AF552987

Duck Rearing and Health Management

NIPA® GENX ELECTRONIC RESOURCES & SOLUTIONS P. LTD.
New Delhi-110 034

Duck Rearing and Health Management

Gunjan Das, M.V.Sc., Ph.D.
Professor & Head
Department of Veterinary Medicine
College of Veterinary Sciences & Animal Husbandry
Central Agricultural University
Jalukie, Peren, Nagaland, India

Mritunjay Kumar, M.V.Sc., Ph.D.
Associate Professor
Department of Veterinary Medicine
Bihar Veterinary College
BASU, Patna, India

NIPA® GENX ELECTRONIC RESOURCES & SOLUTIONS P. LTD.
New Delhi-110 034

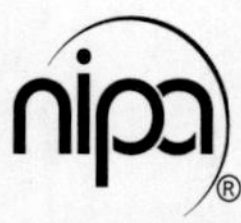

NIPA® GENX ELECTRONIC RESOURCES & SOLUTIONS P. LTD.

101,103, Vikas Surya Plaza, CU Block
L.S.C.Market, Pitam Pura, New Delhi-110 034
Ph : +91 11 27341616, 27341717, 27341718
E-mail:newindiapublishingagency@gmail.com
www: www.nipabooks.com

For customer assistance, please contact
Phone: + 91-11-27 34 17 17 Fax: + 91-11- 27 34 16 16
E-Mail: feedbacks@nipabooks.com

ISBN: 978-81-19072-24-8

Composed and Designed by NIPA.

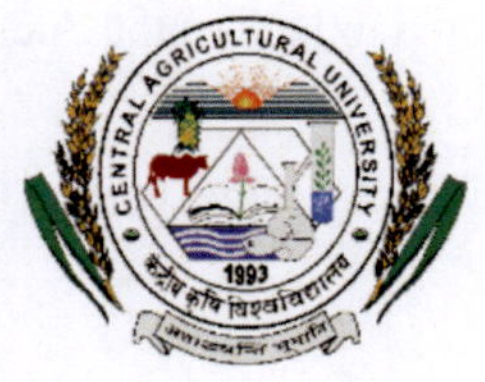

केन्द्रीय कृषि विश्वविद्यालय
लम्पेलपट, इंफाल-795004, मणिपुर (भारत)
CENTRAL AGRICULTURAL UNIVERSITY
Lamphelpat, Imphal-795004, Manipur, India

Tel : (0385) 2415933 (O)
Fax : 2410414
Email : vcofficecau@yahoo.in

No. SVC/CAU/182/2022
Imphal, the 23rd Nov, 2022

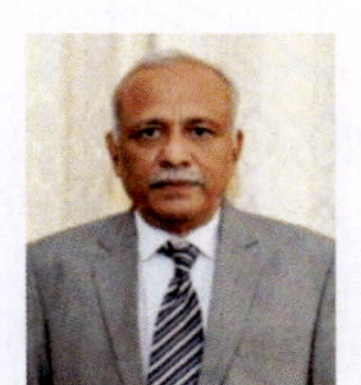

Dr. Anupam Mishra
Vice-Chancellor

Foreword

It is a great pleasure to review the book entitled **"Duck Rearing and Health Management"** prepared with an intention of having a comprehensive handout on duck. Poultry industry of our country is one of the fast-growing sectors of which duck farming plays an important role. Duck rearing is only seen in some parts of our country and has not been taken up as an entrepreneurship in a large scale. Duck are being reared as backyard venture by the small and marginal farmers for meat and egg purposes. It provided livelihood security to many rural households. Duck rearing, duck husbandry and duck health management are very important pillars of duckery.

Ducks play an important role as part of the poultry industry worldwide. There are 1.15 billion ducks worldwide and of which 1.0 billion ducks are in Asia i.e. 88 percent (FAO, 2017). The major proportion of duck populations are found in China, Vietnam, Bangladesh, and Indonesia. Poultry industry is India is one of the fastest growing sectors with 851.81 million poultry population (20th livestock census); of which 33.51 million are ducks. There is 42.36% increase in duck population as compared to 19th livestock census indicating an increase demand of duck meat and egg.

It is really relevant to point out that our institutions have largely depended on the books written by foreign authors based on the information pertinent to their region and countries. It is therefore apparent that a sincere effort is made by the Indian authors to benefit the students and duck rearers from Indian perspective. Moreover, there are very limited numbers of books written on duck rearing and their health management. This book is prepared primarily with an idea of providing an insight into the housing, feeding, nutritional and health management of duck for the veterinary students and duck farmers of this country.

This book comes with 14 informative chapters which are expected to benefit the duck farmers, students, small entrepreneurs and veterinarians.

Let me sincerely compliment the authors for their effort in bringing out this book for catering to needs of the veterinary students, duck farmers, and veterinarians.

Prof. Anupam Mishra
Vice-Chancellor

Preface

The book with a title of **"Duck Rearing and Health Management"** has been prepared primarily with an idea of satisfying the criteria of the Housing, feeding, nutritional and health management of duck for the veterinary students and poultry entrepreneur of this country.

Ducks are sturdy, prolific and disease resistance in nature. In India ducks are reared on natural scavenging system in backyard by poor rural farmers for their livelihood. Ducks are reared for egg, meat and feather production and in India ducks are concentrated in Eastern, North eastern and Southern states of the country. Though ducks' meat and eggs contribution in providing high-quality nutritional food but the production of meat and duck eggs is still lower as compared to chickens. They feed on like insects, snails and waste from kitchen, paddy grains and weeds as natural sources, yet extra feed supplements also need to be provided for better production.

We would like to thank the contributors of various chapters for their timely diligence in preparing the chapters so informatively. We are really indebted to them for their untiring contribution while preparing this First edition, which is the backbone of the book.

The manual is divided in various chapters (Housing, feeding, nutritional and health management etc.). Under health management, infectious and non-infectious diseases are dealt with elaborately. Within each chapter, diseases are listed alphabetically apart from an index, which will further help the reader to quickly locate the required information. I hope our students and readers shall always appreciate the various tables and figures pertaining to the contents. Different photographs pertaining to the breeds and several managemental aspects have been duly presented in places where they are required.

We hope that this book might be an eye opener with regard to the obtaining of good information about the Duck rearing and their health management.

Gunjan Das
Mritunjay Kumar

Contents

List of Contributors

Editors

Gunjan Das, M.V.Sc., Ph.D.
Professor & Head, Department of Veterinary Medicine
College of Veterinary Sciences & Animal Husbandry
Central Agricultural University, Jalukie, Peren, Nagaland, India

Mritunjay Kumar, M.V.Sc., Ph.D.
Associate Professor, Department of Veterinary Medicine
Bihar Veterinary College, BASU Patna, India

Contributing Authors

M. G. Jayathangaraj, M.V.Sc., Ph.D.
Professor & Head, Department of Veterinary Clinical Complex
College of Veterinary Sciences & Animal Husbandry
Central Agricultural University, Jalukie, Peren, Nagaland, India

T. K. Dutta, M.V.Sc., Ph.D.
Professor & Head, Department of Veterinary Microbiology
College of Veterinary Sciences and Animal Husbandry
Central Agricultural University, Aizawl, Mizoram. India

Bikas Chandra Debnath, M.V.Sc., Ph.D.
Assistant Professor, Department of Animal Nutrition
College of Veterinary Sciences and AH, R.K. Nagar, Tripura, India

Tapan Kumar Das, M.V.Sc., Ph.D.
Assistant Professor, Department of Instructional Livestock Farm Complex
(Animal Nutrition), College of Veterinary Sciences and AH, R.K. Nagar, Tripura, India

Bhabesh Mili, M.V.Sc., Ph.D.
Assistant Professor, Department of Veterinary Physiology & Biochemistry
College of Veterinary Sciences & Animal Husbandry, Central Agricultural University, Jalukie, Peren, Nagaland, India

Nibash Debbarma, M.V.Sc., Ph.D.
Assistant Professor, Department of Livestock Production Management
College of Veterinary Sciences and AH, R.K. Nagar, Tripura, India

Imtiwati, M.V.Sc., Ph.D.
Assistant Professor, Department of Livestock Production Management
College of Veterinary Sciences & Animal Husbandry, Central Agricultural University, Jalukie, Peren, Nagaland, India

Lalchawimawia Ralte, M.V.Sc., Ph.D.
Assistant Professor, Department of Veterinary Parasitology
College of Veterinary Sciences & Animal Husbandry, Central Agricultural University, Jalukie Peren, Nagaland, India

Sanjeev Kumar, M.V.Sc., Ph.D.
Assistant Professor, Department of Veterinary Microbiology
Institute of Veterinary Sciences and Animal Husbandry, Siksha-O-Anusandhan (Deemed to be University), Bhubaneswar, Odisha, India

1

Introduction

Domestication is the most extensive biological experiment ever undertaken by man. It has involved millions of animals and has extended through many centuries. It still continues and animal domestication was one of the major contributory factors to the agricultural revolution during the Neolithic period, which resulted in a shift in human lifestyle from hunting to farming. There are two species of domestic duck, the common duck, domesticated from the wild mallard (*Anas platyrhynchos*), and the Muscovy duck (*Cairina moschata*). Both are members of the Anatinae. In both species, the same scientific binomial is used for the domestic and the wild forms. Inter-breeding between the two species occurs, but their offspring are infertile. Both species of domestic duck produce eggs and meat and both are valuable on farms and smallholdings for reducing pests.

Mallards (*Anas platyrhynchos*) are the world's most widely distributed and agriculturally important waterfowl species and are of particular economic importance in Asia. China is the major center of duck domestication, with records indicating duck farming in the region dating back to 2,000 years. It is clear that the domesticated duck originated from mallards, and domestic ducks can be classified as meat or eggs.

Duck farming occupy an important position in India. Among various species of poultry, ducks are sturdy and prolific in nature. They form about 10% of the total poultry population in India and contribute about 7-8% of the total egg produced in country. Ducks lay more egg (about 300 eggs/ year) per bird per year than chicken and the size is also larger than hen egg 18-20 grams. Duck farming plays an important role as part of poultry enterprise worldwide. There are 1.15 billion ducks worldwide and of which 1.0 billion ducks are found in Asia alone (88%) as per the FAO report of 2017. Poultry industry is India is one of the fastest growing sectors with 851.81 million poultry population of which 33.51 million are ducks. Duck meat and eggs are consumed by people worldwide. Rural households can depend on duck farming as it is a lucrative livestock industry within the globe due to its egg, meat and feather as they are prolific and more adaptable to free-range system of rearing compared to chicken. Duck eggs are comparatively larger than chicken eggs. If trained properly the rural people can take up duck farming as an important stride for backyard or commercial production which would help them alleviate poverty and have a sustainable livelihood.

The total population of ducks in India is 33.511 million, which is only 3.93% of the total poultry population of the country. In India, the population of ducks in rural areas (95.98%) are more than the urban areas (4.02%). The top ten duck egg producing states of India are West Bengal (51.52%), Assam (10.53%), Kerala (9.96%), Andhra Pradesh (6.24%), Bihar (5.61%), Tripura (4.77%), Jharkhand (3.13%), Manipur (2.09%), A&N islands (1.42%) and Uttar Pradesh (1.11%). The average egg production in ducks per layer per year is 168, i.e., 146 in desi ducks and 190 in improved duck breeds.

In India duck farming as a small-scale venture has been practiced for many years among rural communities for rural livelihood and income. Domestic ducks have served as a source of food and income for people in many parts of the world since time immemorial. Ducks are a source of meat, eggs and down-feathers (for making bedding and warm jackets). Duck meat and duck eggs are good dietary sources of high-quality protein, energy and several vitamins and minerals. Suitable duck breeds or varieties need to be developed for rural backyard duck farming. Scientific management practices should be adopted to reduce labour input and clean egg and meat production. There is a need for establishment hatcheries and other infrastructures to promote duck farming at rural level for sustainable livelihood of the people.

Prospects and limitations of duck farming in India

Duck form about 10% of the total poultry production in India and also contribute about 7-8% of the total egg produced in the country, opportunities in duck husbandry is enormous viz., self-employment and sustainability that comes with duck farming.

1. Ducks have the natural tendency of foraging on aquatic weeds, algae, green legumes, earthworms, snails, various types of insects reducing their feed cost. Places with extensive inland watershed areas form an excellent habitat for ducks.

2. Cost of rearing duck is less as compared to chicken, duck egg weights 15-20 g more than the chicken, duck lays egg for longer duration then the chicken.

3. Ducks are hardy, easily brooded and are resistant to many poultry diseases. Thus, cost on medication is also lower in duck rising as compared to chicken.

4. Ducks can adapt themselves with almost all types of environmental conditions. They have reduced mortality rate and usually live longer than chickens.
5. Under organized farming system, cannibalism may be seen in chicken but in duck husbandry cannibalism is absent.
6. Duck farming being highly economical and cost effective, has huge potential to engage women folks and farming communities in duck production for achieving financial freedom among rural communities.

However, every enterprise has its ups and downs, likewise there are certain constrain which can be addressed through this chapter:

1. Duck husbandry is one of the most neglected areas in poultry science. Hence, there is lack of scientific knowledge on duck husbandry practices in India, leading to improper management of duck rearing in India affecting production.
2. Small scale producers thereby uneconomical to adopt scientific management practices.
3. Unlike chicken, duck meat and eggs production and consumption are confined only in certain regions of the country southern, eastern and north east parts of India only.
4. Lack of quality germplasm to entrepreneurs interested in setting up duck husbandry.

The following measures can be taken up by the Government to improve the practice of duck farming in India:

1. Establish training centers for the duck farmers to get in-depth knowledge on scientific duck husbandry particularly in eastern and north east parts of India.
2. Provide financial assistance as loans or subsidies for duck farming and strengthen the existing institute for enhanced production and make available quality germplasm to farming communities across India.

Ducks are generally hardier than other poultry. Ducks are raised under a wide variety of conditions, ranging from a backyard coop for a few ducks to modern housing for large flocks on a commercial duck farm. Ducks adapt well to a wide range of systems of care provided as basic care. Ducks need to be protected from extremes in weather conditions and predators. Although ducks can spend most of their time outdoors, on ponds or in wet areas, they require a clean dry sheltered area where they can retreat. Clean water for drinking, a nutritious diet, adequate light stimulation, and protection from diseases are required by them.

To keep the ducks healthy the following steps are needed-

- Maintain biosecurity.
- Immunize ducks against common infectious diseases.
- Minimize environmental stresses which may cause ducks to become susceptible to infections.
- Duck keepers should take care not to use insect sprays in areas accessible to ducks.

In India duck population is concentrated in Eastern, North eastern and Southern states of the country with leading duck population in West Bengal, Assam, Kerala, Andhra Pradesh, Tamil Nadu, UP, Bihar and Orissa, respectively. West Bengal and Kerala are the major consumer states conventionally as regard to duck egg and meat is concerned.

Ducks can be raised in small or large flocks. A small group of ducks can be raised as a backyard endeavour by family as an additional source of meat or earning which, can be established with minimum investment. On the contrary a higher cost involvement is needed to start larger and commercial duck farming. Domestic ducks are said to have originated from the Mallard (*Anas platyrhynchos*) include the Pekin, Rouen, Indian Runner, Khaki Campbell, Cayuga, Albio, Maya, and Tsaiya. The Muscovy (*Cairina moschata*) ducks are different genetically from other ducks; believed to have originated in South America or Egypt is very good meat quality duck. The sterile hybrids (mule) of Muscovy male and common female are popular in some part of the world for lean meat. Duck is also reared for their egg for human consumption and some people have special preferences for the duck eggs. Breeds like Khaki Campbell and Indian Runner most egg producing breeds with approximately 230 to 300 eggs per year.

Ducks are reared under different system of rearing viz. free-range system, confined system and indoor system. In the free-range system, ducks are let loose for the whole day and night shelters are provided. Under confined system, ducks are retained in close place with access to water bodies. Under indoor system of rearing, ducks are reared as a large and commercial purpose. There are other approaches of duck farming also viz. integrated duck farming with agriculture and duck farming with fish and agriculture. Ducks are able to sustain and grow to maturity on relatively simple diets, based on locally available feedstuffs.

Housing, breeding, nutrition and health management of ducks are of utmost importance as regards to the duck farming is concerned. Ducks require a shelter or enclosure with provision of water for their activities. Apart from that a proper housing would protect them from the sun, rain, cold and snow, predators. The shelter is preferred on a high and well-drained area of the backyard having sandy soil as it drains fast after a rain. The sheltered floor should be bedded with straw and dry absorbent material. The housing must be clean, dry and adequately ventilated. Ducks kept on ponds may obtain part of their food from plant and animal in and around the pond. The reproductive performance of ducks is regulated by the length of daylight. Lighting programs generally use a combination of natural daylight and artificial lights to stimulate and maintain egg production and fertility in breeder flocks. Effects of selection of duck, considering egg parameters, controlled growth, exposure to photoperiod, season and suitable conditions for duck egg hatchability are of paramount importance for breeding of duck. A Duck farmer's success mainly depends on source and quality of duck ration which accounts for the major share of the cost of duck production. Feed represents around 65-70% of the total cost of duck production. Therefore, it is to be kept in mind that efficiency in feeding is one of the critical factors for successful duck production. Ducks are very sturdy birds and seldom suffer from diseases as compared to chicken and turkey. They are also resistant to endoparasites unlike their counter parts. However, therapeutic health management along with control and prevention of diseases must be an important aspect of profitable and successful duck farming.

2

Duck Breeds and Varieties

The term "Poultry" indicates to all the domesticated species of birds like chicken, ducks, turkeys, Japanese quail, guinea fowls, geese, pigeons, ostrich, emu etc. Ducks account for 7% of poultry population and are mostly found in coastal states of the country and in states with more lakes and rivers like West Bengal, Orissa, Andhra Pradesh, Tamil Nadu, Kerala, Assam, Jammu and Kashmir and Tripura. Duck farming is still in primitive stage and indigenous ducks outnumbered the exotic ducks in spite of their inferior performance.

In India 90-95% of ducks are indigenous or nondescript types, which are hardly, with mediocre egg production and highly suitable for extensive system of rearing.

Indigenous Duck Breeds/Varieties

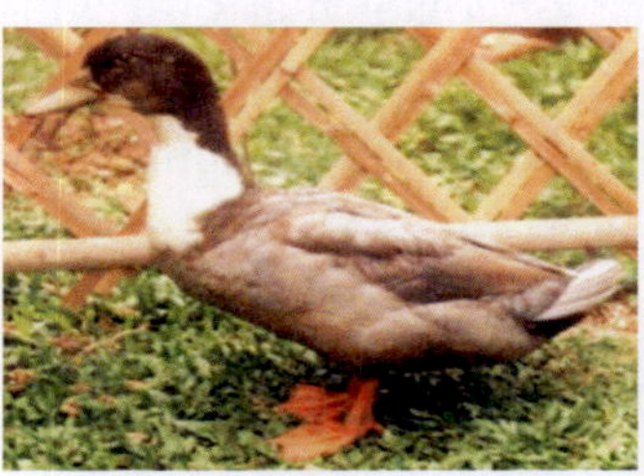

Fig.1 : Nageswari Drake

1. Sylhet mete duck
2. Nageswari (Nagi) - Barak Valley, Assam
3. Pati - Brahmaputra valley, Assam
4. Cina hanh-Muscovy duck, upper Assam
5. Raj hanh - Geese
6. Deo hanh - White winged wood duck, upper Assam
7. Arani - Tamil Nadu
8. Kuttanad - Kerala,
   a. Chara
   b. Chemballi
9. Moti Hansa - Cina hansa, Kalahandi district, Orissa
10. Orissa duck-
    a. White
    b. Khaki
    c. Blue & white
11. Indian Spotbilled Duck
12. Indian Runner Duck.

Nageswari Duck

- Origin: Assam, India
- Age at sexual maturiy-170-205 days
- Egg production is 130-160 eggs.

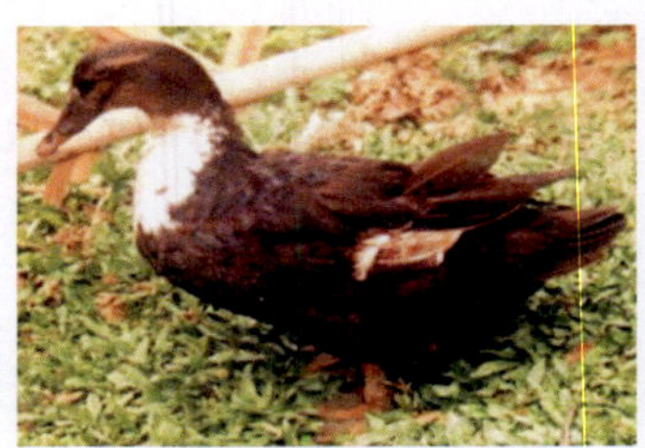

Fig. 2 : Pati Duck

Pati duck

- Origin: Upper Assam, seen in Brahamaputra valley
- Also called as Pati hanh
- Good forager, hardy with higher survivability rate in rural condition
- Nondescript plumage, legs are too short leads almost their body touch the ground which makes them difficult to travel long distance.
- Age at sexual maturity 240 daysEgg production is 80/ year, good sitter

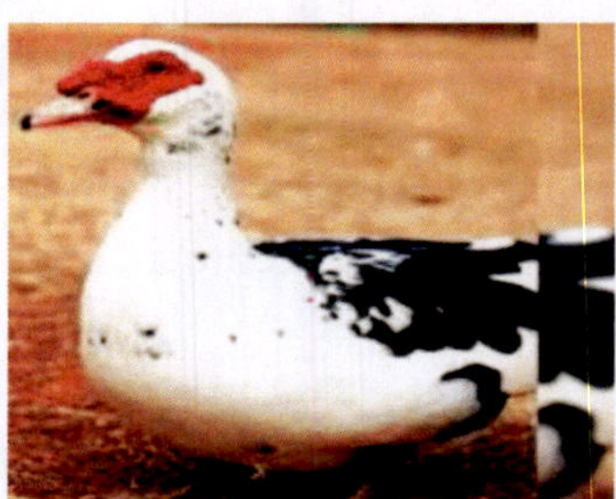

Fig. 3 : Cina hanh duck

Cina hanh duck

- Origin: Assam
- It is a Muscovy duck also called as Bor china or Bhatt china
- Ornamental bird with unique tuft feather on the head
- Age at sexual maturity 290-325 days
- Egg production 45-65 eggs.

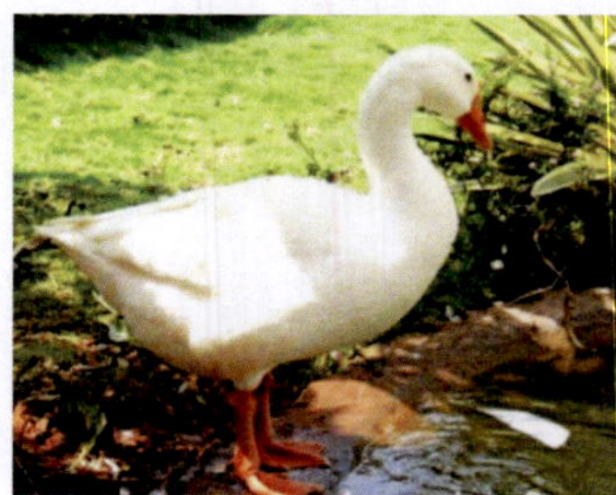

Fig. 4 : Raj hanh (Geese)

Raj hanh (Geese)

- Origin: Assam
- Ornamental bird
- Age at sexual maturity 320-355 days
- Egg production 25-35.

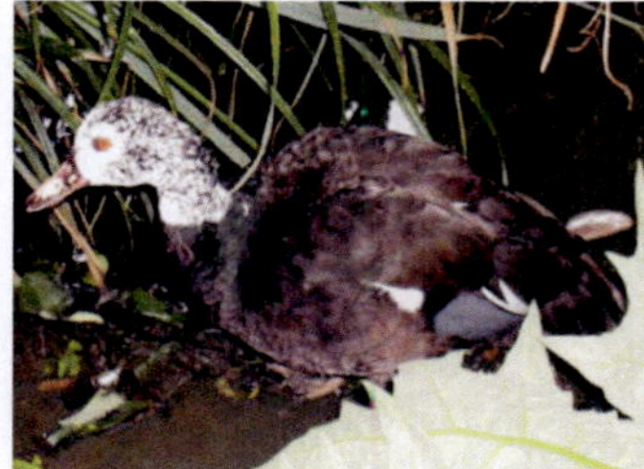

Fig. 5 : Deo hanh (White-winged wood duck) (Geese)

Deo hanh (White-winged wood duck)

- Deo hanh (*Cairina scutulata*)
- Origin: Assam, India
- Commonly called as White-winged wood duck, Cachar, Hagrani & Daophlantu
- Scientific name: *Cairina scutulata* (Muller, 1842)
- Wild duck having delicious meat quality

Aarani ducks

- Originated from Aarani taluk, Thiruvannamalai district, Tamil Nadu.
- Sanyasi – It is named due to its dull brown colour as base colour throughout the body.
- Drake – It is upright in posture & gait; Plumage colour is dull brown with or without white patches; Neck – lustrous blackish green with or without white bands; Shanks & bill – dark orange.
- Duck - Squat in posture & gait; Plumage colour is dull brown with or without white patches; Neck - dull brown with or without white bands; Shanks & bill – dark orange.
- Weight (20 wks) Drake 1.582kg Ducks 1.543kg

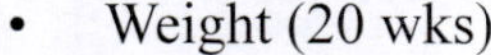

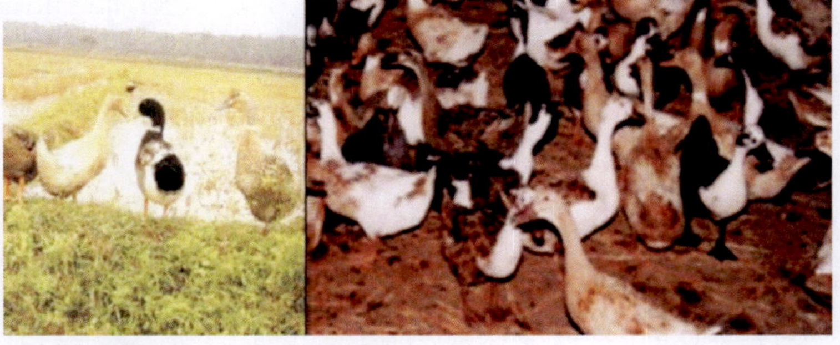

Fig. 6 : Aarani ducks (Geese)

- Keeri - Named after its plumage pattern, blackish brown stripes in the base of brown color.
- Drake - Upright in posture & gait; Neck-dull blackish green; Body colour-brown with blackish brown stripes all over the body; back-predominantly blackish brown; Shanks & bill are orange.
- Duck - Squat in posture & gait; plumage-brown with blackish brown stripes; Shanks and bill are orange.
- Weight (20wks) Drake 1.559kg Ducks 1.511kg
- Egg production - 160-200 white eggs.

Chara duck (Kuttanad Ducks of Kerela)

- Chara duck is named based on plumage colour.
- Drakes are squat in posture and gait.
- Head - lustrous greenish black, neck is longer (21.1cm) in drakes than ducks (18.7), is brownish black with full or half white band on the front

of neck. The breast plumage is brown & brownish grey. 'Wing speculum' (two dark areas on both side of the body and is covered with black feathers) present.

- Bill (7.0cm) - dull orange with black spots; feet-bright orange.
- Ducks head, back & tail are blackish brown; breast-brownish black but light brown and white are also observed. Female is more nervous.
- Bill (6.02cm)-shorter than male, yellowish black, yellow with black spots or yellow in colour.
- Weight (at 20wks) Drake 1.643kg Duck 1.538kg
- Egg production 180 - 200 white shelled eggs.

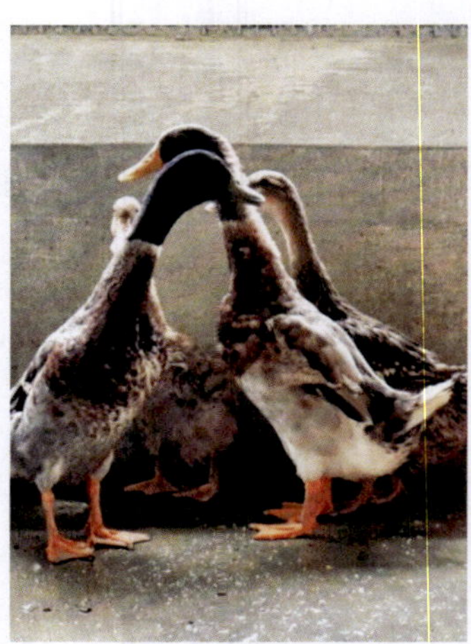

Fig. 7 : Chara duck (Kuttanad Ducks of Kerela) (Geese)

Chemballi duck (Kuttanad Ducks of Kerela)

- Named based on their plumage colour.
- Drakes are squat in posture and gait.
- Head dull greenish black; neck is longer in drakes (21.07cm) than ducks (18.95cm), has brown plumage with full or half white bands; back & tail covers-brownish black; wing feathers are brownish grey, primary & secondary feathers are light and deep brown mixed with white and rest of body light brown plumage. Wing speculum present.

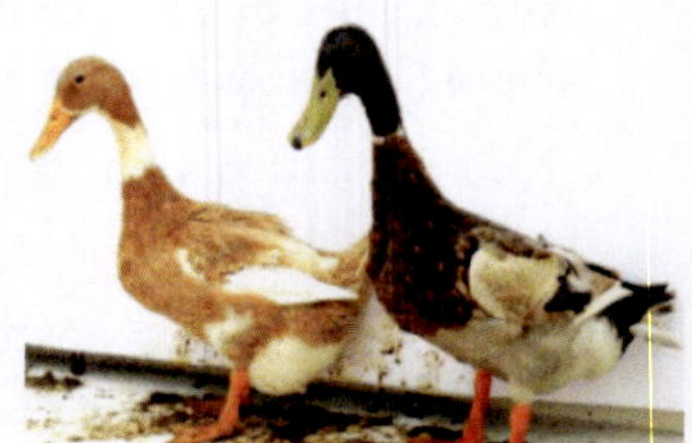

Fig . 8 : Chemballi duck (Kuttanad Ducks of Kerela)

- Bill is longer (7.0cm) in drake than duck (6.03cm), yellow with black spots.
- Feet are bright orange in colour.
- Ducks little squat in posture.
- Plumage is brownish black and brownish grey in back, tail and wings, wherein brown is predominant over black and grey.
- Head-brownish black; neck-brown with or without white band; back & tails covers-brownish black; wing feathers-brownish grey with primary

and secondary are light & deep brown mixed with white; breast-light brown and brownish black.

- Bill is yellowish black, yellow with black spots or yellow.
- Feet are dull orange.
- Weight (at 20wks) Drake 1.658kg Duck 1.498kg
- Egg production 180-200 white shelled eggs.

Moti Hansa

- Muscovy duck in Kalahandi district, Orissa (Imported by olden Kings from South America).
- Also called as Naka hansa, Kudi hansa or Cina hansa
- Used for table purpose, rarely for eggs by tribal people.

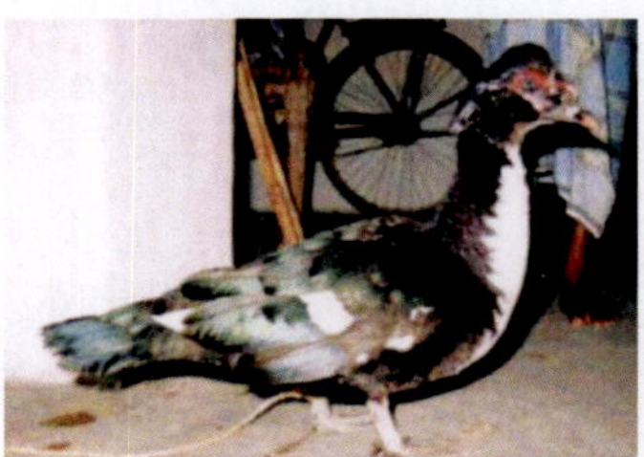

Fig. 9 : Moti Hansa (Geese)

- Head - fairly large, flat at top and larger in males; Crest present in both sex; Head width 31.86 - 41.56; Caruncles are fairly large and found in both sides of face and eyes.
- Bill - short, fleshy tubercle at base of bill.
- Plumage - Mixed white, brown, white & brown, brown & black, white & black and black & blue; black plumage in wings changed to white during 2nd year.
- Weight Drakes 3.5 kg Ducks 2.56 kg
- Egg production 50 – 60 eggs.
- Broody, fairly resistant to stress and worm infestation.

Orissa Duck Breed

- Habitat: Koraput, Malkangiri, Nawarangpur, Nawapara, Kalahandi, Mayurbhanja & jagatsinghpur districts of Orissa
- Also called as Koraput White duck, Koraput Khaki duck etc.
- Light class bird, dual purpose, sensitive (flyaway for slight disturbance)
- Back - Parallel to ground, alert, active and have pleasing appearance
- Head - Round, slender & proportionate to the body
- Bill - Yellow in white variety and light grey to dark grey in other varieties. Bill of drake is larger than duck

- Eyes - Round & blue in white variety and black or brown in other varieties
- Neck small, widest at base & tapers down towards the head; a distinct white lone separates the neck from body in Koraput Khaki ducks
- Body small & round, back is uniformly flat, longer than width; breast is wider in males; abdomen in longer in females
- Wings - Medium in size, placed close to body, colour is similar to body colour
- Skin - White to yellow in colour
- Tail - Small, carried to the same level of back & colour is similar to body colour
- Shank is smaller, shank is longer is male; shank colour varies according to age, becomes dark orange /yellow in adult
- Weight Drake 1.5-2.2 kg Duck 1.3-1.5 kg
- Egg production 100-130 white shelled eggs.

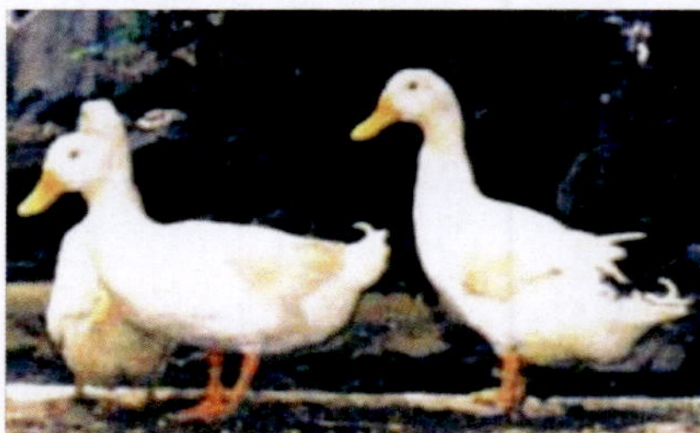

Fig. 10 : Orissa White Duck (Geese)

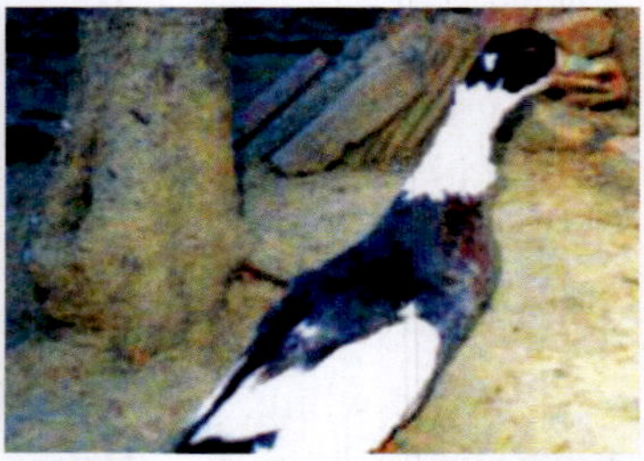

Fig. 11 : Orissa Blue & White duck

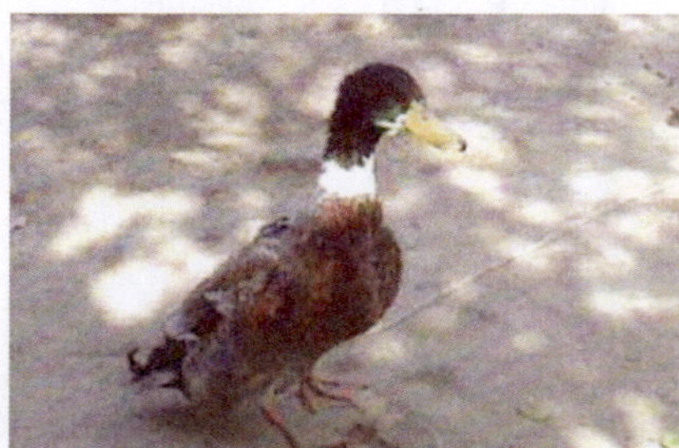

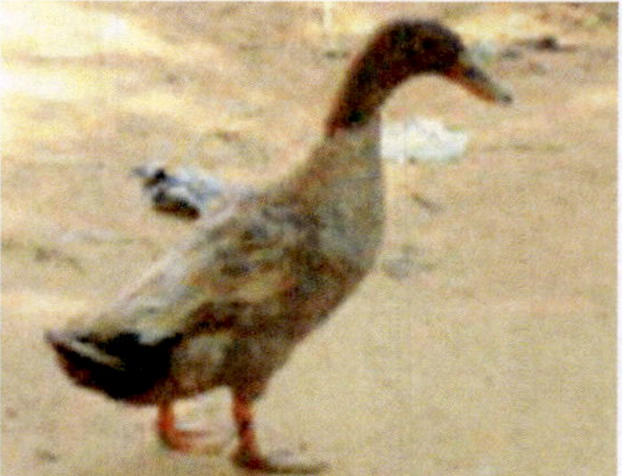

Fig. 12 : Orissa Khakki duck

Sylhet Mete Duck

- They are found mainly in eastern India.
- Major part of the body is covered by light brown feathers with black tip, but the head and neck are blue.

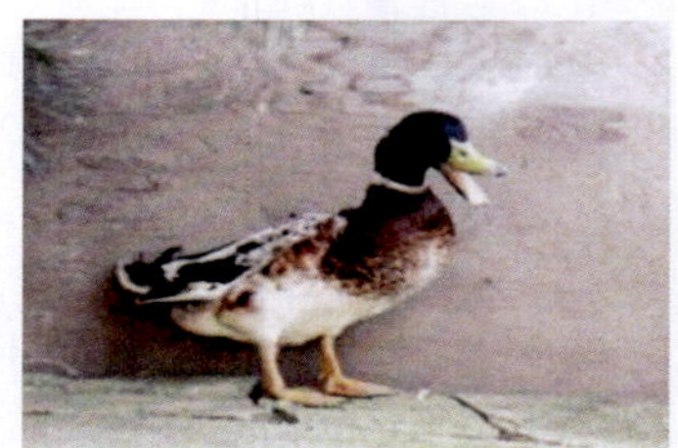

Fig. 13 : Sylhet Mete Duck duck

- The number of eggs produced per year is 80-150.
- The average weight of white shelled egg is 56gm.
- The weight of a fully grown bird is about 1.8 kg.

Indian Runner Duck

- They are also called as "penguin ducks" because of their upright body posture.
- They're considered as "light class "domesticated duck breed as their flesh to bone ratio is high.
- They produced around 300 to 350 eggs per year.
- Their body colour ranges in white, brown and blue.

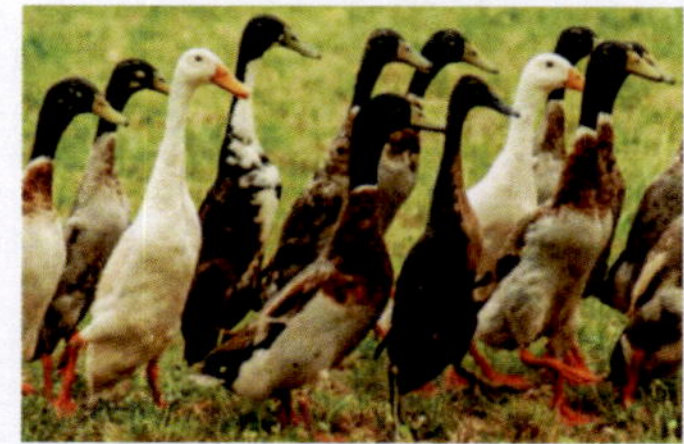

Fig. 14 : Indian Runner Duck duck

- Adult female ducks weigh around 3 to 4 lbs and adult drake weigh about 3.5 to 5 lbs.

Important Points about Ducks

1. Scientific name of duck is *Anas platyrynchos*.
2. Chromosome number of duck is 40 pairs.
3. Incubation period of duck is 28 days.
4. For duck age at sexual maturity is 28-30 weeks.
5. Ducks are classified into 3 types as Egg production, Meat production, Ornamental purpose type as per as their utility.
6. Male adult duck is known as drake & female adult duck as duck.
7. Ducks are more prolific and produces 15-20 eggs more than backyard chicken.
8. Size of the duck egg is 10-15 gram larger than chicken egg.
9. Ducks have long productive and profitable life *i.e.,* they will lay in second and third year also.
10. Ducks supplement their feed by foraging; hence it will reduce the feed cost.
11. Marshy, swampy river side, wet lands, barren lands not suitable for chicken can be used for duck rearing.
12. Ducks lay their eggs during early in the morning (3 am to 8 am) and saves time and enables easy egg collection.

13. Duck farming is having symbiotic relationship with paddy cultivation, so ducks and paddy cultivation can be integrated in the entire paddy farming areas.
14. Ducks are quite intelligent birds and they can be easily trained for their daily routine (going to ponds, feeding etc.) and it reduces the labour for management.
15. Ducks are quite hardy; ducklings are easy to brood and are resistant to common avian diseases.

3

Housing Management of Duck

Duck farming in India is characterized by nomadic, extensive, seasonal, and is still held in the hands of small and marginal farmers. Traditionally Assam, West Bengal and Kerala are the major consumer states for duck egg and meat and one of the reasons is that duck egg and meat highly suits and impart taste for their fish based culinary preparations.

Different housing system for Duck rearing

In general, ducks do not require elaborate houses. The house should be well ventilated, dry, and rat proof. In semi-intensive system of rearing, the house should have easy access to outside run as the ducks prefer to come out during the day time, winter and rainy time. The run should have slope away from the house to provide drainage. In the house of semi-intensive system, a continuous water channel of size 50 cm wide and 15-20 cms depth should be constructed at the far end, on the both sides, parallel to the pen in the grower and layer house.

The houses for ducks are designed to protect them from extreme weathers, parasites, predators and thieves to avoid the development and spread of infections, contagious disease and to facilitate the labours and attendant to work efficiently. Housing accounts most of the cost in the poultry farming so the veterinarian should have the full knowledge about the different housing system of duck to save unnecessary land wastage in building and sheds.

Location of a Duck Farm

Farm should be located in the area where there is good market for eggs and duck and at the same time labours and rations should be readily available at cheaper rates The farm should be well connected with roads and other modes of transportation. Electricity and water should be available at reasonable cost and ease. Farm should not be constructed in a cities or near residential areas where it is objectionable or prohibited by law because it may not be possible to shift or dismantle permanent buildings on legal notice or objections. It should be located away from the crowded areas and should have enough space for future expansion. As far as possible the farm should be away from disturbances like noise, vibrations, Pollution etc.

Factors Influencing Design of Houses for Duck

Designing a building involves a series of compromise between ideals and feasibility to give best economic performance. Following are the main factors to be considered:

- Temperature.
- Ventilation.
- Humidity.
- Floor, feeder and water space requirement
- Light
- Orientation of house.

Temperature

Ducks being warm blooded (homeothermic) poultry have the ability to maintain their body temperature. The mechanism (homeostasis), however, is efficient only when the ambient temperature is within certain limits; birds cannot adjust well to extreme weathers. Therefore, it is very important that ducks be housed and cared for, so as to provide an environment that will enable them to maintain their thermal balance.

Ventilation

Proper ventilation requires the movement of fresh air into the building and removal of stale air out of the building in such a way to produce a healthy atmosphere in all parts of the house.

Humidity

Correct humidity is another important factor for efficient performance of ducks in the shed at different stages of life. High humidity in sheds is very harmful to ducks and it may help in the development of pathogenic microorganisms causing diseases in birds. Low humidity in houses result in dry and dusty litter and this might lead to respiratory ailments. So, the relative humidity in the house should range between 40 to 60 per cent.

Requirement of floor space, feeders and waterers

The requirements for floor space vary according to age, size and type of birds to be maintained. The requirement with respect to these are given in tables 1-

Table 1: Space requirement of adult duck under different system

Intensive system	Semi- Intensive system	Free range system
2-2.5 sq.ft area per duck	3 sq.ft.per duck	No definitive space requirement

The brooding period of layer ducklings is 3-4 weeks while for meat type ducklings 2-3 weeks. During chilly season, brooding period needs to be extended by 1-2 weeks longer than the regular period. Hover space of 90-100 sq.cm per duckling may be provided under the brooder. A 200-watt bulb can brood 30-40 ducklings. Under wire floor system of brooding, the space recommended is 0.5 sq.ft per duckling. Under deep litter system; it is 1.0 sq.ft per bird up to three weeks of age. Water in the drinkers should be 5.0-7.5 cm deep, just sufficient to drink and not to dip themselves.

Grower (5-16 weeks)

Ducks can be reared both in intensive and semi-intensive system. Under intensive system, floor space of 3 sq.ft per bird up to 16 weeks of age is sufficient. Under semi intensive system of rearing, a floor space of 2-2.5 sq.ft per bird for night shelter and 10-12 sq.ft per bird for outside run is necessary for free flow of birds up to 16 weeks. Water in the drinkers should be 10 -12 cm deep to allow the immersion of their heads.

Layer (above 17 weeks of age)

Under intensive system, a floor space of 4 sq.ft per bird is essential. In semi intensive system a floor space of 3 sq.ft per bird for night shelter and 10-12 sq.ft per bird of outside run space is required. For wet mash feeding 10 cm of feeding space and for dry mash or pellet feeding 7.5 cm of feeding space per bird is required.

Orientation of House

The effects of weather elements are strongly directional. Orientation of a building with respect to wind and sun consequently influence with force, precipitation, temperature, and light on different external surfaces. Where there is freedom of space, it is expedient to orient buildings to achieve the maximum control over the microclimate. The broad face of a house obviously endures greater wind pressure than does that narrow dimension under the same wind speeds. This may be desirable if high temperatures are prevalent, but it becomes problem if winds are exceptionally vigorous or cold.

The rules which govern the relation of sunshine to site exposure apply equally to building orientation. In the Northern Hemisphere, the greatest amount of insulation is received by the east and southeast sides of a house in the morning and by the west and southwest sides in the afternoon. In summer, with increasing latitude, the path of the sun in the sky describes more complete circles so that the sun rises north of east and sets north of west; in winter they are of the sun's visible path is shortened, and east and west exposures receive very little sunlight. Ordinarily, an east-west alignment of a rectangular house provides the maximum gain of solar energy in winter and minimum in summer.

Light in poultry house

The visible light is only part of the radiant energy spectrum which falls between 400 to 700 mm. Ducks appear to see better when the illumination is through long end of the spectrum, otherwise they behave similar to man and have colour visions. Light intensity is expressed in "foot candle" (f.c.). A bulb at 2.1 m from the floor surface, 1 watt of power for 0.55 sq. m. surface area will give an intensity of 1 f.c. with tungsten light and 3.6 f.c. with fluorescent light.

There are two factors influencing the intensity of light falling on birds: (1) power of light source, the amount of light given out by the bulb is directly proportional to its wattage and (ii) distance of surface from the light source. The light intensity decreases as the source of light is placed farther away from the surface.

In most of the tropical countries laying and rearing houses have over 1/4 of wall area open as windows and doors and it may not be possible to exclude natural light below critical level where there is no physiological response of the light on birds. Hence, it is difficult to reduce the day length in the sheds below the natural day length. Day length longer than this natural can be provided with extra supplementation of artificial light during dark hours.

Day length varies throughout the year and hence the performance of birds is also expected to vary accordingly. Ducklings hatched during March-April will be getting increased day length during its growing period leading to an early sexual maturity, lower body weight. smaller and fewer eggs throughout their laying period.

A conditioning period of 4 to 6 weeks of short-day length of 8 hours or as followed by 3 weeks of long day length of 15 to 17 hours are needed before the egg production is desired. The intensity and colour of light may be similar as for chickens. But in practice, a light intensity of 1 to 2 f.c. of white tungsten bulb is given.

Method of providing light- Light in poultry shed should be evenly distributed. The ratio of light from poorly lit corner to brightly lighted corner should not be more than 1:3, i.e., if poorly lit corner has light intensity of 1 f.c. the bright area should not have more than 3 f.c. In case, this ratio becomes wider than the birds in brightly lit area are likely to develop cannibalism. Such uneven distribution of light will lead birds to utilize only comfortable area of the shed. Both poorly and brightly lit areas will remain unutilized.

Poultry Houses

Depending upon the activity on poultry farms following buildings may be needed. One type of building may be used for other purposes depending upon the requirement. Like a brooder house can be used as broiler house or even as a layer house. Following buildings related to poultry farming will be discussed in this chapter.

- *Hatchery*
- *Brooder House*
- *Grower House*
- *Layer House*
- *Poultry processing unit*
- *Feed Mill*

If more than one type of houses is to be constructed on one farm, these buildings should be located in such a way that it cuts down the chances of cross contamination to minimum, affords maximum labour efficiency and better supervision of farm with least effort.

Hatchery

It is a place where artificial incubation of eggs is undertaken for production of chicks/ducklings. The size of hatchery can vary from a few hundred eggs capacity to several million eggs. The hatcheries are classified on the basis of size, kind of ducklings/chicks they supply, sources of hatching eggs to hatchery etc.

Location: Preferable a hatchery should be located in the area where there is demand for ducklings/chicks and availability of good transport facilities. It has been seen that some of the successful hatcheries are located at the far distance from actual users. Sometimes this is advantageous to check the cross infections from farm to the hatchery.

Building: A hatchery can be located in any type of building available with certain amount of success. It may range from a spare farm house to well designed and constructed hatchery building. Little can be said for the buildings to be adopted except that the requisite equipments will have to be fitted in as best as they can be. Even for specially designed hatchery there cannot be a universal blue-print because the size and shape of incubators vary for the same capacity, area, topography etc. However, there are some general principles that can be offered as guidelines for those who are interested in construction and operation of a commercial hatchery.

A well-designed hatchery can be divided in two parts -

i) Administrative side - It includes offices to keep the records and deal with correspondence and orders. These offices should be well lit and comfortable for efficient working of staff. If the hatchery is sufficiently large, a separate enquiry office with a telephone may be necessary. A waiting room for the visitors and customers may be provided with a display unit showing the working of the hatchery, advertising its products, and providing a supply of advertising literature.

ii) "Work" Side - It may have the following rooms or sections: Receival platform, room for traying of eggs, egg cleaning and washing room, fumigation chamber, dark room, incubator and hatcher room, sexing, packing and dispatch rooms, washing and sterilizing room for equipment, stores and such other ancillary accommodation as generator room, service room and garage and waste disposal room. All rooms should be located in orderly manner which involve minimum travel and avoid cross infection of diseases.

Egg Receival: The egg receiving room should be directly accessible to the road way and must be large enough to store large number of egg boxes full or empty. It should be such that it can be closed when the eggs are detained for overnight with the help of collapsible shutter. There may be a stand with writing facility for keeping records of incoming eggs and the date of setting and incubator used etc.

Egg Traying Room: Egg traying may be done on a permanent rack or it may also be done on trolley which can be moved around to fumigation chamber and then to incubator when the eggs are to be disinfected. Out of these two, use of trolley is recommended and they should have pneumatic tires to avoid vibration when moving.

Fumigation chamber: Eggs are fumigated before setting. It will be connected with egg reception and traying room preferably with concrete and tiles so that trolleys are pushed in and out easily. A pipe of 2 cm internal diameter can be fixed to the wall so that formalin can be added to potassium permanganate after room be closed. The same pipe can also be used to pour ammonia to neutralize the excess formaldehyde when fumigation is over. This room should have air tight doors and a power aided extractor ventilation system discharging gas direct to outer air. It is an advantage to ventilation is by forced draft intake, with the outlet covered by hanging lovers so bad that they are closed when the fan is not working and opened when fan is working to move the gas.

Incubator Room: It should be well connected with other rooms of "work" side by means of sliding doors wide enough to allow easy handling of trolleys. Actual shape of the incubator will be dictated by the size, make and number of incubators to be used. A thumb rule is that 5.5 cu m space for every 1,000 eggs incubated. The ceiling height should not be less than 3 m. To ensure good ventilation there should be at least 0.5 m distance from the walls and incubator frame. Ventilation in this room should be adequate. Minimum of eight circulation of air in the room per hour should be enough. Draft should be avoided. For efficient working of machine and persons working in this room, temperature of 21.1°C may be maintained by providing a heating or cooling system.

A separate hatching room has an added advantage in reducing the incubator spread of diseases and in maintaining high level of hygiene. A separate hatching room should have tight fitting for doors and ventilators and if possible, should be provided with separate ventilation system.

Sexing Room: It should be connected with incubator room and hatcher room if it is a separate section in one side and packing room on the other. This room should be warm (24°C), well ventilated and should have shelves to hold chick boxes. The sexing table should have metallic top or may be plastic covered so that it can be washed often. Each table must be equipped with high powered overhead light which is adjustable for height. Cleanliness is of the vital importance in sexing.

Packing and Dispatch Room: It should have adequate bench space and racks, and should be connected with sexing room on one side and roadways and delivery window on the other. It should also have the space to accommodate empty chick boxes and place for recording.

Washing Room: Good facilities are required for washing and scrubbing incubator fittings, trays and trolleys. The washing room needs fairly large tanks in which various fittings can be soaked, scrubbed and rinsed.

Store Room: It should have ample space to store chick boxes, packing materials, spare incubators fittings, labels and several other things. It should be well planned with respect to racks, lighting and connected with hatchery.

Other facilities needed at the farm may include a stand-by power generator room, bath and washing rooms for male and female employees etc.

The landscaping around hatchery should be made as attractive as possible. Customers are to apt to associate quality of the chicks produced with appearance of the building and environment in hatchery.

Brooder House

Most of the layer or broiler houses can be used efficiently as brooder house. However, there are some advantages and disadvantages of having a permanent brooder house.

Advantages

1. The house can be used throughout the year for brooding since it is designed to aid temperature control both in cold and hot weathers.
2. Less labour is required for the care of young flock.
3. Less problem, of disease contamination from old to young stock.

Disadvantage

The investment on permanent brooder house is relatively high and often a separate brooder house is not fully utilized throughout the year.

The design of brooder house depends upon the system of brooding practice. There are two systems of brooding (i) Floor brooding and (ii) Battery brooding. Floor brooding is further divided into two types, namely, hot room and cold room brooding. The later one is more commonly used in tropical countries.

The floor-cum-battery brooder house has proved satisfactory under north-western arid zone of India and likely to be suitable in other parts also. Both floor and battery brooding can be one in this house. When brooding is not done, the brooding pens can be utilized for rearing of replacement pullet or broilers.

Battery room can be used starting chicks for flock replacements, for broiler production, for holding surplus chicks from hatchery or for feeding experiments etc.

Processing plant

There are several considerations need to be given in designing a processing plant like construction, cost, size of the business, facilities for personnel, equipment, layout and ease of maintenance etc.

Most of the plants have eight general work areas. These are receiving, hanging and slaughtering area, defeathering, eviscerating, packaging refrigeration room and shipping or disposal area. In addition, storage areas, offices, toilets, lockers for workers, machinery rooms and refuse rooms are considered as auxiliary areas.

Building should be constructed so as to prevent the entrance of flies and rodents by providing properly fitted screens or other suitable devices. The floors, walls, ceilings, partitions, posts, doors, etc. should be constructed of materials with a hard and smooth finish which can be readily and thoroughly cleaned. Slope and construction of floor in the areas where water spills like scalding, defeathering, evisceration and chilling should be such that water drains off without making slippery floor. The pitch should be 1cm per meter to the drains. Water supply should be pure and ample. Building should be well ventilated and lighted. There should be provision for washing equipment, hands and utensils.

Layer House

Ducks are able to adjust to a wide range of environmental conditions as indicated earlier but they perform well at any temperature up to 30°C in a dry, well-ventilated house free from ammonia, dust and air-borne pathogens. The business becomes profitable when ideal environmental conditions are accompanied with labour saving devices in the house so that it involves minimum walking for gathering of eggs, feeding and watering of birds.

There are four types of layer houses used in intensive system of duck rearing (Deep-litter housing, Cage system, Slat system and Slat cum litter system). In Deep litter system of housing, the ducks are kept on floor in a building in which they are free to roam about. The floor is covered with litter of sawdust, straw or any such materials and they have a run area provided with a channel of water. The advantages of deep-litter system over the cage system are:

- Less investment.
- Less difficulty in fly control.
- Offers the advantage of self-control of birds during extreme weathers.
- Less labour involved in collection and handling of eggs
- Litter as source of fertilizer.

A distance of 30 m to 45 m should be provided in between two laying sheds to minimize the chances of infection and fire hazards.

The following points should be considered while deciding for a plan of layer house -

i) ***Size of house***: It depends upon the size of flock to be maintained and the area needed can be calculated at the rate of 2300 sq cm to 2800 sq cm per bird but it is suggested that the unit should not be bigger than to accommodate 500 birds.

ii) ***Width of house.*** Under tropical conditions a poultry shed should not be wider than 9 m. It is more desirable to limit the width to 7.5 m. In case of wider house, birds tend to remain towards the periphery of the house and the central part of the shed is less efficiently utilized unless forced-draft ventilator is installed.

iii) ***Partition.*** Partitioning of large house should be done to accommodate 500 to 1000 birds. In a bigger flock culling of poor and sick birds and overall control is difficult whereas labour cost decreases per bird. In a smaller flock culling and supervision are easier but the attendant has to enter in a greater number of pens to take care of the birds.

A thumb rule which usually works well is to keep the length of pen 1.5 times more than the width. A 6 m wide house should have the pens of 6 x 9 m.

iv) ***Height of ceiling.*** During summer, much of radiated heat can be reduced by keeping the ceiling at higher level, but in no case, it should be less than 3 m. A ceiling at 3.5 m is more desirable where summer is severe.

General construction of laying house

After deciding the plan of the laying house, detail blue-print should be made with the help of qualified architect or house builder showing every detail of the shed. Following information may be of some use where the help of experienced qualified personnel is not available.

Foundation- It should have enough hold on the ground to support the building. Most permanent poultry houses have concrete foundations. The depth at which the foundation ditch should be dug for foundation walls will depend on the height of the house, kind of soil and the need to keep out the rats. Forty-five cm deep and about two times wider than walls, foundation is dug. The earth from foundation may be used to increase the level of floor.

Floor- The floor should be strong and non-yielding. The floor may be either of cement concrete or brick laid in cement mortar or stone slabs set in cement mortar or 'kaccha' floor made or dirt, sand and gravels. The 'Kachcha' floor is difficult to disinfect. Eight to ten centimeters thickness of well-mixed concrete (1 part concrete, 2 parts cement and 4 parts gravel) laid on well tamed base is usually sufficient. The floor should be 0.25 m higher than outside surrounding elevation.

Walls- The lower portion of the walls up to the height of 0.6 m should be of solid brick and masonry work. The upper portion of the walls may be made of chicken wire mesh supported by brick masonry pillars of 30 x 30 cm spaced along the outside of the side walls and ends of supporting the rafters and roofs. The frame netting of chicken wire mesh should be made of angle iron or wooden-frame depending on availability and cost.

Rafters, girders and roof- The rafters and girders are used to support the roof. Type and spacing depends on the kind of roof used. For asbestos roofing, girders of 5 x 15 cm are set on the edge of the posts for supporting roof. Rafter of 5 x 10 cm is spaced about 0.6 m apart on the girders to fasten the roof.

The roof may be lean to gabled type- In case the width of house is more, gabled type roofs recommended. The roofing materials may be of asbestos cement sheet, aluminum sheets, galvanized iron sheets or thatch. The metallic roofs are hot in summer and cold in winter. These are durable and become cheap in long term. Thatch roof provides good insulation and is cheap in winter unless used with insulation like thatch etc. In case of metallic roofs, the upper surface should be painted with white aluminium paint to reflect sun rays and a wide overhang should be provided to protect the house from wind, rain and sun.

Cage house

There are certain advantages and disadvantages of cage system which should be given due consideration before, deciding about the cage system of poultry rearing.

Some of the advantages are like easier culling, less problem due to parasites, predators and other diseases since the birds do not come in contact with litter. Large number of birds can be kept in a limited space as well as uniform and clean egg production throughout the year etc.

The pitfalls of cage housing which should be kept in view are higher housing and equipment cost per bird; increased labour requirements; odour and fly problems. A better environmental control and well-balanced feed are needed under cage system since birds need to adjust according to the changes of environment and feed conditions; cage fatigue also is one of the important problems encountered under cage system of rearing birds.

Common arrangement of cages

During early thirties, 3-deck laying cages were popular in U.S.A. but slowly trend has come for single deck cages largely because of convenience in working.

Single deck cages may be in lines of cages facing to the central aisle of cage house or back cages in lines with several aisles in a cage house.

The other type of arrangement of cage is double deck arrangement which is not common and may be considered where it is necessary to increase the housing capacity and where environmental temperature is low and there is need to utilize body temperature of birds to keep the house warm. Yet another arrangement is off-set staggered or step arrangement. This is also used where poultrymen wish to increase number of birds under a given roof area.

There are mainly three cage systems, namely single bird cages, multiple bird cages and colony cages where in each cage 20 to 30 birds are kept.

Cage housing. The cage houses seem to work satisfactorily in sub-tropical areas. It works ideally where day and night temperature do not go beyond 32°C and -4°C for long time. The cost of operating cages goes up beyond the above temperature range.

South and coastal parts of India appear to be most suited for cage housing where temperature fluctuation is not much and remains, moderate throughout the year. But in north and western parts of the country, summer and winter become severe. Therefore, a wide variety of housing designs ranging from completely open from sides to well protected side walls having arrangements for opening and closing windows depending upon weather will have to be considered.

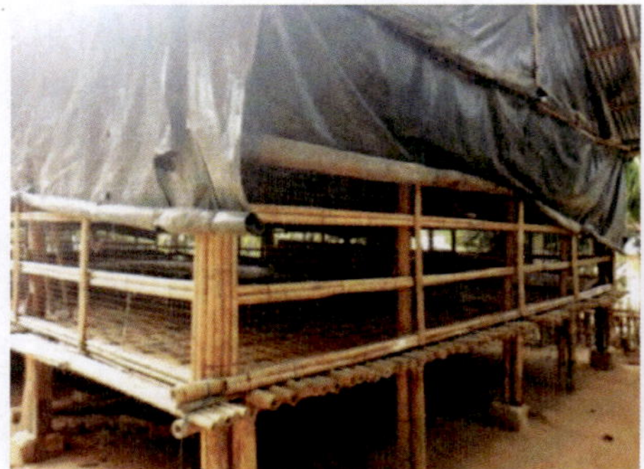

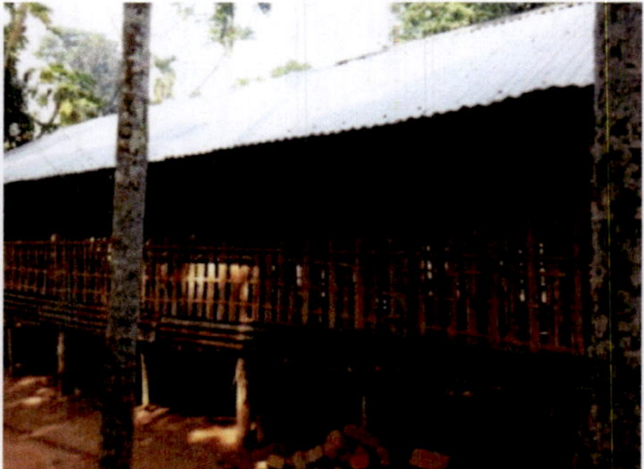

Fig. 1 : Duck housing with bamboo wall and bamboo floor

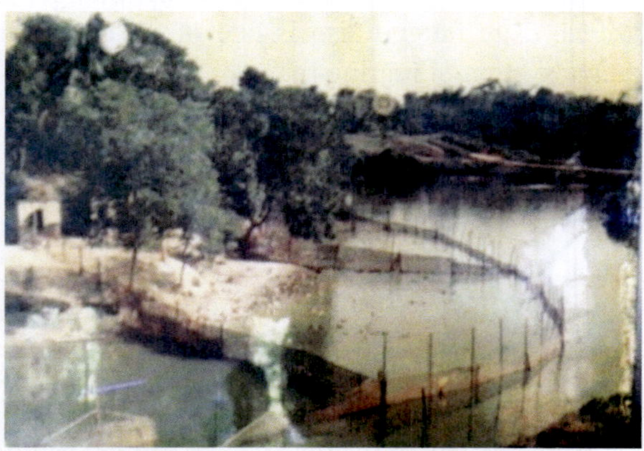

Fig. 2 : Ideal traditional duck housing in coastal/ wet land

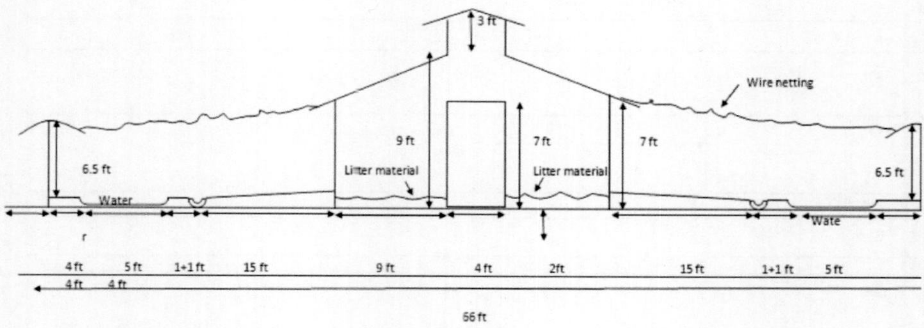

Fig. 3 : Duck house layout plan for 400 layer/ 600 Grower (Cross-sectional view)

A	4 ft
B	5 ft
C	1 ft
D	15 ft
E	9 ft
F	4 ft
E	9 ft
D	15 ft
C	1 ft
B	5 ft
A	4 ft

Where:
A = Resting Area, B = Water area, foot dip, C = Gutter, foot dip, D = Feeding area,
E = Laying area, F = Middle passage

Fig. 4 : Detail floor layout for 400 layer duck/800 grower duck

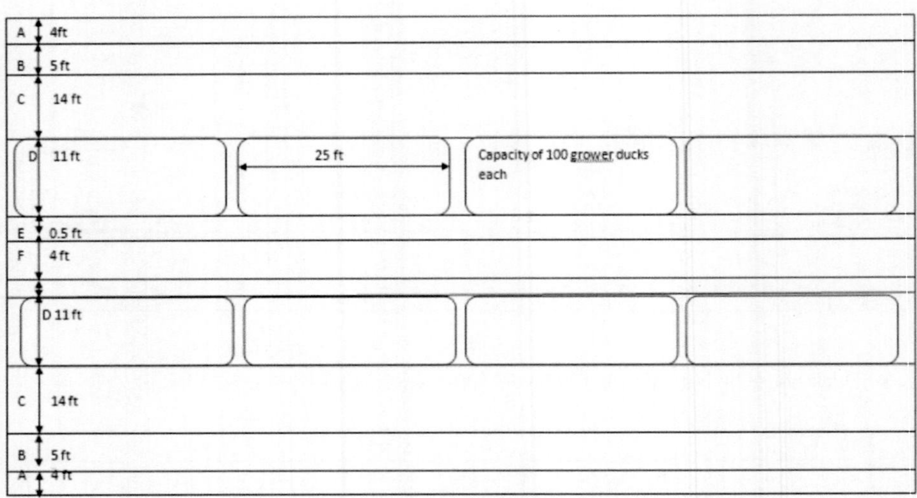

Where:

A= Resting area, B= Water area, foot deep, C= Feeding area, D= Lying area, E= Gutter, 0.5 foot deep, F= Middle passage

Fig. 5 : Detail floor layout plan for 800 grower duck

References

Ajit Kumar, (2021): Duck farming: a profitable source of income to farmers. Just Agriculture 2 (2): 6-8.

Bais (2014). Poultry line, May, pp.27-31.

Jha BK. Chakrabarti a (2017). Duck farming: a potential source of livelihood in tribal village. J.animal. Health. Prod. 5(2): 39 & 40

Makram, A. 2016. Ducks world. In: proc. 9th Intl. Poultry Conf. Nov 7-10

Msa Bhuiyan, Ds Mostary, Ms Ali, Mm Hussain and Ajm Ferdaus 2018 performance of Nageshwari ducks Bangladesh Journal of Animal Science 46(3):198

N.S.R Sastry and C.K.Thomas (2014): Duck farming Prod. Manag. Pract.. Reg. Cent. Centl. Avian res. Inst., Bhubaneswar, pp: 1-31

Panda (2005). Guidelines for duck farming. Reg. Cent. Centl. Avian res. Inst., Bhubaneswar. AJAS,8 (4):375-378.

Prafulla Kumar Naik and Bijaya K Swain (2022): Scenario of duck population in India Poultry Line, pp 25-27

Purabi Kaushik, Jnyanashree Saikia, Kabitabala Kalita, Rajjyoti Deka 2021: Morphology and morphometry characteristics of pati duck. Int. J. Chem. Stud., 9 (1):351-354.

Rajesh Singh (2020). Diagnosis, treatment and control of nutritional deficiency disorder in poultry, Pashudhan Praharee, December 26

Rolandsossinka (1982). Domestication in birds, Avian Biology 6,373-403.

Sastry and thomas 2015: Livestock production management pp 694,710.

Zebin zhang, yaxiongjia, (2018): whole-genome resequencing reveals signatures of selection and timing of duck domestication. Gigascience (7)1-11.

4

Indigenous Ducks of India and Their Physiological Parameters

Duck (*Anas platyrhynchos*) is one type of indigenous poultry species, reared traditionally by the poor farmers for their livelihood. Maximum numbers of duck flocks concentrate in the paddy (*Oryza sativa*) growing and watershed areas of the state like Assam, Bihar, Manipur, Kerala, Andhra Pradesh, Tamil Nadu, Orissa, and Tripura. Ducks rise on the free-range system with readily available fallen grains in paddy fields, insects, snails, earthworms, small fishes, and other aquatic materials. The available ducks are a few eaotic breed (khaki campbeel, whitepekin) and locally available indigenous or non-descriptive breeds (Pati, Maithili, Nageswari, Chara, Chemballi etc.). Indigenous or non-descriptive breeds are relatively better resistant to common diseases, require lesser attention, and thrive well in scavenging conditions. The baseline physiological and haemalo biochemical values are vital for health care management with a thorough physical examination under scientific duck farming. Therefore, this chapter discusses the overview of the baseline physiological values of Indigenous ducks of India.

Physiological parameters

The resting body temperature, heart rate, and respiratory rate of ducks range 106-108°F, 180-230 breaths/minute, and 13-40 breaths/minute, respectively. These values vary with size, body weight, age, recent activities, health status, and environmental condition. The high body temperature of ducks enables them to keep on warm even when the temperatures are below freezing.

Erythrocytic parameters

Erythrocytes in the circulating blood of ducks are nucleated like chickens. The key function of erythrocytes is the transport of oxygen. The average length of the erythrocytes is 5.668 µm to 16.049 µm, and the width ranges between 3.750 µm to 10.115 µm. The life span of erythrocytes is 30 to 40 days. The short life span of erythrocytes in ducks may be due to their high body temperature and metabolic rate. The reference value for erythrocytes parameters of duck is given in Table-1. The factors like genetics, breed, sex, age, body weight, seasonal factors, health staffs, etc affect the erythrocytes values. Duckings have 100 TEC, which progressively, mineares with advancement of ages. The higher TEC in adult bird in due to The mineased level of androgens than young ones erythrocyte counts contribute to the information for the diagnosis, surveillance, and formulation of a prognosis regarding the future progression of a disease in an individual.

Leucocytic parameters

Leucocytes/ white blood cells are motile cells in the blood. These cells help the body fight against infection and other diseases. Types of leukocytes are heterophils, eosinophils, basophils, monocytes, and lymphocytes (T cells and B cells). The number of leucocytes is far less than the number of erythrocytes. The reference value for leucocytes parameters of duck is given in Table-1. The factors such as infection, environmental conditions, stress etc affect the leucocyte counts. A complete blood count (CBC) includes the hemogram, which contributes valuable information in the differential diagnosis of a particular disease or pathological condition and detecting the effects of environmental, parasitic, infectious, or toxicologic stresses on individuals.

Table 1: Mean hematology value of Ducks.

Sl. No.	Parameters	Indian Runner		Muscovy		Indigenous Ducks	
		Male	Female	Male	Female	Male	Female
	TEC ($\times10^6$ μL^{-1})	2.69±0.18	1.90±0.10	2.06±0.22	1.99±0.28	2.62 ± 0.03	
	PCV (%)	35.70±2.85	33.60±2.91	36.40±3.67	34.60±2.89	50.00± 0.69	
	Hb (g/dL)	13.91±0.20	10.05±1.05	12.69±1.08	12.00±0.78	10.39 ± 0.14	
	MCV (fl)	192.27±19.36	129.71±13.52	228.42±49.71	192.27±19.36	172.29 ± 1.39	
	MCH (pg)	54.33±6.56	53.41±3.00	66.43±5.79	54.33±6.56	59 88 ± 2.3	
	MCHC (pg)	28.90±2.51	44.96±4.69	38.94±5.81	28.90±2.51	39.46 ± 0.75	
	TLC ($\times10^3$ μL)	9856.00 ±1720.92	9541.40 ±1594.03	14072.90 ±2331.26	14071.00 ±2593.86	10.92 ± 0.21	
	Basophils (%)	1.70±0.44	1.70±0.47	4.70±0.20	3.90±0.58	-	
	Eosinophils (%)	7.40±2.51	9.30±3.93	29.80±3.38	16.60±3.91	1.22 ±0.10	1.29 ± 0.11
	Heterophils (%)	38.80±7.01	40.10±6.47	12.90±2.70	25.70±8.74	58.85 ± 0.39	58.20 ± 0.53
	Lymphocytes (%)	46.80±5.71	43.70±5.3	38.50±2.44	38.50±4.10	30.40 ± 0.38	31.30 ± 0.53
	Monocytes (%)	14.10±1.30	15.30±2.10	5.30±1.82	5.20±1.33	9.65 ± 0.27	9.40 ± 0.34

TEC: Total Erythrocytes count; TLC: Total Leucocytes counts

Blood Biochemical parameters

Normal blood levels of various biochemical constituents are indispensable for normal body functions and productive performances. Glucose is the primary metabolic fuel required for vital organ function, growth, and performance. Total protein, Blood Urea Nitrogen (BUN), and albumin are useful indicators for assessing protein status. Urea nitrogen concentration is influenced by wide variety of interrelated parameters *viz* dietary protein intake and rumen degradability, dietary amino acid composition, protein intake relative to requirement, liver and kidney function and muscle tissue breakdown.

Liver enzymes most frequently looked at for health issues include Aspartate Aminotransferase (AST), Alanine Aminotransferase (ALT), and Alkaline Phosphatase (ALP). ALT is found primarily in the liver; AST is also found in skeletal muscles and erythrocytes. These enzymes level elevates by a high-fat, high-protein diet, weight gain, changing exercise levels, disorders including liver disease, and other physiological and environmental causes.

The baseline biochemical value of the Indian duck breeds is given in Table-2. The variation in the mean serum biochemical's value of ducks is due to genotypes, sex, reproductive status, egg-laying, level of nutrition, and geographical location. The serum biochemical profile contributes information about weight gain, metabolic disorders, general health status, and effects of environmental effects on ducks.

Table 2: The serum biochemical profile of different Duck breeds of India.

Sl. No.	Parameter	Pati variety duck	Khaki Campbell duck	Nageswari duck
	Total protein (g/dL)	5.84±0.19	6.83 ±0.22	5.93 ±0.16
	Glucose (mg/dL)	145.69 ±10.12	159.78 9.23	171.62 ±7.63
	Albumin (g/dL)	4.05 ±0.10	5.52 ±0.19	3.95 ±0.12
	Globulin (g/dL)	1.79 ±0.10	1.31 ±0.10	1.98 ±0.09
	BUN (mg/dL)	1.27 ±0.06	1.23 ±0.12	1.65 ±0.22
	Uric Acid (mg/dL)	4.51 ±0.11	4.15 ±0.09	4.44 ±0.22
	AST (Units/L)	75.20 ±4.29	75.25 ±3.60	64.17 ±4.15
	ALT (Units/L)	22.01 ±0.29	21.65 ±0.28	29.51 ±0.31
	ALP(Units/L)	86.44 ±4.29	86.56 ±6.51	91.25 ±7.15

The baseline information about the physiological parameters, hematology, and serum biochemical value of indigenous ducks serves as a guide for assessment growth, health status, routine herd investigations, and monitoring. However, each laboratory should establish a set of reference intervals of hematology and serum biochemical values according to a defined series of steps to rule out the geographical and environmental effects on it.

References

Acharya C P., Bhattacherjee A, Mallik B K. and Mohanty P K. Int. Res. J. Biological Sci. 8 (9), 8-16. 2019.

Bhattacherjee A, Acharya C P, Rana N, Mallik B. K. and Mohanty P. K. Comp. Clin. Pathol. 27, 1465–1472. 2018.

Friendship R M and HenryIovasculr S C 1992. In: Leman, A. D., Straw, B.E., Mengeling, W. L. D'Allaire, S., Taylor D. S. eds. Disease of swine. 7th Ed. Iowa State University Press, Ames AI. pp.3-11.

Kalita D J, Bezbaruah N and Barkakati J. The Pharma Innovation Journal. SP-9(4): 36-38. 2020.

Kavitha K, Raj Manohar G, Vairamuthu S and Ramamurthy N. International Journal of Science, Environment 5: 4, 2621-2624. 2016.

Mili B, Pandita S, and. Parmara M S. Livestock Research International, 3(2): 43-46. 2015.

Rat, R, Panigrahi B, Mishra S K, Pradhan C R, Maity A. and Tewari H. Indian J. Anim. Res.53 (3), 327-331. 2019.

Roland L, Drillic M. and Iwersen, M. J. Vet. Diagn. 26(5): 592-598. 2014.

Spano J S, Pedersoli A W M, Kemppainen B R J, Krista B L M. and Young D. W. Avian Diseases 31:800-803. 1987.

Sujatha C, Jayanthy, N.R. Kumar S, Sunder J, De A K, and Bhattacharya, D. Indian J. Poult. Sci. 56(2): 149−153. 2021.

Swathi B and Sudhamayee KG. Indian J. Poult. Sci. 40 (2): 146-149. 2005.

5

Nutrient Requirements of Ducks and Their Feeding

Duck production has an immense role in improving the socio-economical status of rural farmers. In India, duck farming occupies an important place next to chicken farming. Duck contributes about 7-10% of the total poultry population of the world. Ducks are water fowl, hence, they need a semi-aquatic lifestyle. They need a pond, lake, river, canal or any such type of water bodies for their survival. Thus, they are mainly concentrated in West Bengal, Assam, Andhra Pradesh, Orissa, Kerala, Tripura, Tamil Nadu, Bihar, Jammu & Kashmir and Manipur. Ducks are reared for both eggs and meat purposes. Unfortunately, duck farming is not done in an organized way in our country.

A Duck farmer's success mainly depends on source and quality of duck ration which accounts for the major share of the cost of duck production. Feed represents around 65-70% of the total cost of duck production. Therefore, it is to be kept in mind that efficiency in feeding is one of the critical factors for successful duck production.

Advantage of duck rearing

- Growth rate of duck is fast. The feed conversion efficiency is 3-3.5.
- Laying ducks lay 250-300 eggs per year.
- Feeding costs of duck can be reduced to some extent as they are voracious eaters of forages.
- Water bodies are normally utilized for rearing of ducks.
- Ducks like to eat compounded feed. Apart from this, they eat snails, slugs, finger-lings, earth worm, insects and vegetation. Hence, feed cost can be reduced to a great extent.

There are various breeds of ducks found in India. Among them some of are good producers. Indian Runners, (white and fawn) and white and Khaki Campbell are good breeds for egg production. They weigh between 2-2.5 kg.

Khaki Campbell Duck

It is an egg laying breed. Khaki Campbell is the best egg producer. They are originated by crossing a Malaysian Indian Runner female (duck) with a Ruen male duck (drake). They lay 250-300 eggs per year. Khaki Campbell ducks weigh about 2 to 2.2 kg, and drakes 2.2 to 2.4 kg. Egg size varies from 65 to 75 g.

Pekin Ducks

It is originated from China. The Pekin ducks are found to the most popular meat type duck for table purpose in the world. White Pekin ducks are broiler type. In 8 weeks of rearing their body weight become 3.3-3.6 kg with a feed consumption of 9.6-9.9 kg. It is fast growing and has low feed consumption with fine quality of meat. It attains about 2.2 to 2.5 kg of body weight in 42 days of age, with a feed conversion ratio of 1:2.3 to 2.7 kg.

Vigova Super-M broiler duck

It is a cross between White Pekin duck and Aylesbury duck produced in Vietnam. This breed was imported by the Central Duck Breeding Farm (CDBF), Hessarghata, Bangaluru from Vietnam. The ducks weigh 3 kg at 49 days of age.

Digestive System of Ducks

The anatomy of digestive system in the duck is a peculiar one because the system is different from that of chicken. The ducks do not have beak instead of it they have a peculiar structure called bill. They also lack teeth. The bill can easily separate feed mixed in water. Due to their bills it becomes difficult to take submerged food material as well as consumption of the most dry mash food particles of appropriate size. Other small peculiar structures are present which border the outer margin of the tongue and upper and lower bill is called papillae. Most of the dry mashes form a sticky paste when mixed with their saliva and stick on to these papillae and other structures bordering the outer margin of the tongue. Such sticky paste interferes with the movement of the food materials to the tongue which may choke and results in reduced feed intake and increase in feed wastage when the duck tries to shake or wash off the mash materials adhering to the mouthparts. The lower part of its mouth is not stiff or rigid so it can flex out to some extent to allow the duck to obtain food particles. Food is taken into the esophagus. Unlike other birds, the ducks do not have crop. Due to absence of a crop the ingesta passes very quickly which is actually quicker than the other poultry birds. From the esophagus, the food enters into a thin-walled cylindrical structure of the glandular section of the stomach called the proventriculus. The proventriculus is connected to the muscular structure known as the gizzard. The gizzard leads into the small intestine. The pancreas is located on the small intestine. The small intestine leads into the large intestine which leads into the caecum and then colon. The colon empties into the cloaca through which waste products are excreted. The gallbladder is located within the lobes of the liver and bile duct connects the gall bladder to the intestine.

Digestion of Carbohydrates in Duck

The digestion of carbohydrates starts at the mouth cavity and ends in the small intestine.

- Digestion in the mouth cavity: Saliva is secreted from the salivary gland. Saliva has two digestive enzymes. One is ptyalin or salivary amylase and another is maltase. Ptyalin acts on boiled starch only and maltase enzyme on maltose. Ptyalin does not act on uncooked starch; it acts only on boiled starch. Ptyalin converts boiled starch to maltose.
- Digestion in the proventriculas: No carbohydrate splitting enzyme is available in the gastric juice. However, HCl of gastric juice has some ability to hydrolyze some sucrose to glucose and fructose.
- Digestion in the intestine: Bile has no carbohydrate digestive enzymes. Pancreatic juice has two carbohydrate digestive enzyme viz. pancreatic amylase and maltase. Pancreatic amylase acts on both boiled and unboiled starch. So, boiled or unboiled starch and dextrins are digested to maltose by pancreatic amylase enzyme. Maltose is digested to glucose by maltase enzyme. Digestive juices of succus entericus for carbohydrate digestion are sucrase, lactase, maltase, isomaltase, α-limited dextrinase and intestinal amylase. Sucrase converts sucrose to glucose and fructose. Lactase converts lactose to glucose and galactose, maltase converts maltose to glucose, isomaltase converts isomaltose to glucose, α-limited dextrinase converts alpha limited dextrins to glucose and intestinal amylase which is present in minute amount digests boiled or unboiled starch to maltose.

Absorption

Absorption of monosaccharide may result by either passive diffusion or active transport. Fructose, mannose and other pentoses are absorbed passively. Glucose and galactose are absorbed by active transport which requires energy and Na+. Rate of absorption of hexoses; galactose has the highest followed by glucose and fructose. The rate of absorption of carbohydrates by bird is rapid. Feed passes rapidly through the digestive tract.

Digestion of Proteins in Duck

Digestion of protein starts at stomach and ends at small intestine.

Digestion in the stomach

- There are two proteolytic enzymes present in the stomach viz. pepsin, gelatinase.
- Proteins like albumins, globulins, etc. digested to peptone by the enzyme pepsin (proteins - acid metaprotein - primary proteose - secondary proteose - peptone). Pepsinogen is the precursor of pepsin.
- Nucleoprotein is digested to nuclein by the enzyme pepsin.
- Mucin is digested to glucosamine and peptone by the enzyme pepsin.
- Gelatin is converted to gelatin peptone by the enzyme gelatinase.

Digestion in the small intestine: Bile has no proteolytic enzyme.

Digestion in pancreatic juice: The proteolytic enzymes of the pancreas are *trypsin, chymotrypsin, aminopeptidase, tripeptidase, dipeptidase, carboxypeptidase, ribonuclease, elastage, collaginase*, etc.

- Trypsin is the precursor of trypsinogen which converts proteins or peptone to lower peptides or amino acids.
- Aminopeptidase converts polypeptides to amino acids.
- Tripeptidase converts tripeptides to amino acids.
- Dipeptidase converts dipeptides to amino acids.
- Carboxypeptidases convert polypeptides to amino acids.
- Ribonuclease converts nucleic acid to nucleotide.
- Elastase converts elastin proteins to peptone.
- Collaginase converts collagen protein to peptone.

Digestion in intestinal juices: The proteolytic enzymes of intestinal juices are erepsin, polynucleotidase, nucleosidase, nucleotidase, etc.

- Erepsin converts polypeptides or lower peptides to amino acids.
- Polynucleotidase converts nucleic acid to nucleotides.
- Nucleosidase converts nucleosides to purines, pyrimidines base and pentose, phosphate.
- Nucleotidase converts nucleotides to purines, pyrimidines base and nucleosides.

Symptoms of protein deficiency

Marginal deficiency in duck causes increase in appetite and increased feed intake. In layer chicken marginal deficiency of protein will not cause reduction in egg production but causes the reduction in egg size. But a severe deficiency of protein in the diet of growing chicken causes slow growth, poor feathering, lack of appetite, feather picking and cannibalism. A severe deficiency of protein in layers will cause reduced feed consumption and a marked decrease in egg production.

Symptoms of excess protein intake

A diet having more than 30% protein results in a higher concentration of uric acid in the blood. There is deposition of crystals of calcium urate salts in the soft tissues of visceral organs. Also, there is deposit of crystals in various joints.

Digestion of Fat in Duck

Digestion of fat starts at stomach and ends at small intestine. In saliva there is no splitting enzyme. Neutral fats, phospholipids, cholesterides, etc. are digested in the gastro intestinal tract.

Digestion in the stomach

Gastric *lipase* enzyme is secreted from the stomach which acts in acidic pH i.e. at 4-5. By this enzyme neutral fats are converted to fatty acids and glycerol. Steps in hydrolysis of neutral fats:

Fat------→Fatty acid + diglycerides.

Diglycerides-----→fatty acid + monoglycerides.

Monoglycerides------→ fatty acid + glycerol.

So, in complete hydrolysis of 1 molecule of fat there is production of 3 moles of fatty acids and 1 mole of glycerol.

Digestion of fat in the small intestine

In small intestine fatty foods are mixed up with bile, pancreatic juice and intestinal juice.

Functions of bile: Emulsification of fat is caused by bile salts (sodium glycocholate and sodium taurocholate) through which fat molecules become soluble in water. This emulsified fat is digested by the pancreatic and intestinal juices.

Digestion in pancreatic juices

These gland secrets lipolytic enzymes like *pancreatic lipase, pancreatic phospholipase, pancreatic cholesterol esterase,* etc.

- Pancreatic lipase enzyme is secreted from the pancreas which acts in alkaline pH i.e. at 8. By this enzyme neutral fats are converted to fatty acids and glycerol. Steps in hydrolysis of neutral fats:

  Fat→Fatty acid + diglycerides.

  Diglycerides→fatty acid + monoglycerides.

  Monoglycerides→ fatty acid + glycerol.

  So, in complete hydrolysis of 1 molecule of fat there is production of 3 moles of fatty acids and 1 mole of glycerol.
- By the enzyme pancreatic phospholipase lecithins are digested to fatty acid and lysolecithin.
- By the enzyme pancreatic phospholipase cephalin are digested to fatty acid and lysocephalin.
- By the enzyme pancreatic cholesterol esterase cholesterol ester is converted to fatty acids and free cholesterol.

Digestion in intestinal juices

- Intestinal lipase digests fat into fatty acids and glycerol.
- Lecithinase converts lecithin in to fatty acid, phosphoric acid and choline.

Role of vitamins in duck nutrition

Thiamin: Thiamin is closely associated with carbohydrate (energy) metabolism. Thiamin plays an important role in the transmission of nerve impulses. It is believed that thiamin is required for acetylcholine synthesis. Its deficiency causes paralysis of neck, leg and wing muscles.

Niacin: It is desirable to supplement niacin in the diet of duck ration. Brewer's yeast is the best source of niacin. Tryptophan can replace niacin to an extent of 10%. Ducks do not have the ability to convert trytophan to niacin because they have a 3-4 folds higher level of *picolinic acid carboxylase* than chicken which prevent tryptophan to convert into niacin. So, ducks may be less efficient than chickens in converting tryptophan to niacin. Ducks are more susceptible to bowed leg condition and leg weakness resulting in complete crippling associated with niacin deficiency. Other symptoms include lack of growth, diarrhea and weakness.

Riboflavin: In Riboflavin deficiency, the ducklings fail to grow after 2 or 3 days and usually die within 4-7 days. There appears to be an excess of secretion from the eyes and eyelids may become stuck together. There is a slow growth. There is no report of curled to paralysis.

Pantothenic acid: Its deficiency symptoms are similar to riboflavin deficiency.

Pyridoxine: Severe acute deficiency of this vitamin in ducklings causes failure of growth and severe anemia. Neither convulsion nor paralysis is observed in ducklings. A chronic deficiency in the older ducks causes lack of growth, paralysis, convulsions, severe microcytic anemia and poor feathering.

Biotin: A deficiency leads to very poor growth.

Choline: Its deficiency leads to perosis (slipped tendon).

Vitamin A: Poor hatchability and heavy early mortality, nasal discharge, paralysis, etc. are some common symptoms of vitamin A deficiency.

Vitamin D_3: A deficiency of this vitamin causes rickets in ducklings, soft rubbery bones, rough feathering, poor growth, muscle degeneration, weakness.

Vitamin E: It is a natural (biological) antioxidant at cellular level (protects the lipid structure of phospholipid membrane). It prevents the oxidation of unsaturated fatty acids that is mostly present in all cell membranes. It prevents myopathy of gizzard and skeletal muscles.

Vitamin C: Reduction in the mortality of ducklings and significant increased weight gain are observed on supplementation of vitamin C at the dose rate of 240 mg per liter drinking water.

Role of minerals in Duck nutrition

Copper: Copper supplementation results in increased growth rate and smaller caeca.

Selenium: A deficiency of selenium causes muscular dystrophy in ducks.

Iodine: Supplementation of iodine in the form of iodine causes increased growth rate, feed efficiency, and feathering and reduced carcass fat in ducklings.

Dry mash, wet mash and pellet feeds

Dry mash versus Wet mash

Normal feed ingredients for a poultry ration can be compounded for a duck mash. Dry as well as wet mash can be fed to the ducks. But the problem always arises with the dry mash feed. They face great difficulty in swallowing this dry mash. Whenever they take this dry mash, it forms a sticky paste in the oral cavity as mentioned earlier. So, they will take mouthful and rinse it down in the nearest water body and hence it causes heavy loss of feed nutrients. Thus, the growth performance is reduced by around 10% as compared to the pellet ration. To avert this problem, dry mash should be mixed with drinking water and such wet mash may be offered to the ducks. Usually, wet mashes are offered to the ducklings (up to 2 weeks of age) 4-5 times daily and afterwards it should be 3-4 times daily. So, it is seen that wet mashes need to be given at frequent intervals and after each meal residual wet mash is to be removed. However, dry mash, crumbles and pellets can be offered to the ducks at free choice basis.

Pellet feed

Nowadays pellet feeding has become popular in developed countries. Though pellet feeding is little bit costly, it has distinctive advantages such as saving of feed with least amount wastages, saving in labor, convenience and hygienic conditions improvement. Pellet feeding should be started at two weeks of age. Pellet size of 3.97 mm diameter and 8 mm length is suitable for duckling. A pellet size of 4.76 diameter with 13 mm length is normally preferred after 2 weeks of age. The ducklings showed highest average weight both at 4 and 8 weeks due to pellet feeding. As far as better feathering and general development of duck is concerned, pellet feeding shows better result than mash feeding at 12 weeks age. Pellet feeding showed an excellent result in egg production in the first and second laying year.

Natural Feeding Habits

Ducks are normally voracious eaters. Ducks are good foragers too. A lot of edible feeding materials for the ducks grow in the natural aquatic environment. When ducks are reared in pond, apart from compounded feed they eat seeds and green parts of aquatic plants, snails and other mollusks, crustaceans, finger-lings, earth worm, water insects and vegetation which also reduce the feed cost. These are obtained during diving and from the water surface. In addition to the natural feeding, little amount of concentrate mixture can be offered for a better growth rate and egg production.

Feeding in Intensive Rearing

The ducklings after hatching are reared for four weeks in the brooding house. During this time, they should be properly fed with duck starter ration. The ration should contain adequate energy and protein level (2500 Kcal/kg and 20.5% protein) for their rapid growth. The first eight weeks is very important for the ducklings and they should always have access to feed. Afterwards, they may be fed twice a day i.e. first in the morning and then late afternoon.

Egg type duck breed like Khaki Campbell duck consumes about 12.5 Kgs. of feed up to 20 weeks of age. Afterwards, an adult female duck consumes 170-230 g per day. However, the feed intake may vary depending upon the rate of production and availability of greens. Ducks can be raised on dry or weight mashes. It is better to feed green feeds which can be chaffed and are of good quality like berseem, Lucerne, etc.

Common Feed Ingredients

Cereals and their by-products

Appropriate feeding of duck needs a major portion of the ration includes cereal grains and their by-products. In this regard they contend directly with the human beings for cereal feeding. Cereal comes under family *Graminae*.

Cereals

Maize (*Zea mays*): The chief source of energy in ducks is supplied through maize. Among the cereals, it is the richest source of energy. Maize has a high ME value (3340 Kcal ME/kg). A pigment, cryptoxanthene present in yellow maize is the precursor of vitamin A. Maize has only 8-9% CP) which is also of low quality. The protein is deficient in tryptophan, methionine and lysine. Nowadays, two varieties of maize are available namely Opaque-2 (rich in lysine) and Flury-2 (rich in lysine and methionine). This cereal is very low in CF but has 73% starch on dry matter basis. The egg size of ducks is controlled by lenoleic acid, an important factor in diet. Maize is rich in this lenoleic acid. Inclusion level of maize in duck is 50-60%.

Wheat (*Triticum aestivum*): The palatability of wheat is very high. Normally broken wheat is used for feeding of duck. Its feeding value is better than either oat or barley. CP in wheat ranges from 8-14% (on dry matter basis). Wheat, especially if finely milled, forms a pasty mass in the mouth of ducks which leads to digestive disturbance. Wheat bran, a by-product of this grain, contains 12-14% CP. Wheat contains more of B-complex vitamins than maize. Inclusion level in case of duck is up to 50%.

Rice (*Oryzae sativa*): Rice is highly palatable, digestible and a good source of energy. Normally broken rice is used for feeding of duck. It has a Metabolizable Energy (ME) value of 2845 Kcal/kg. Inclusion level in both ducklings and duck is up to 40%.

Sorghum/ Jowar (*Sorghum vulgare*): Sorghum is quite hard grain due its tough seed coat. Hence, it becomes difficult to digest. Moreover it is slightly less palatable to maize. For mixing with other ingredients, it is used after crushing and grinding. Protein content of sorghum varies from 8.5-12.5%.

Metabolirable energy value is 2645 Kcal/kg. Depending upon the amount of tannin (an anti-nutritional factor) present, there are two varieties of this grain. Inclusion level in duckling is less in dark variety (0-10 %) while in white variety it is 0-25% while it is 0-20% and 0-40% in adult ducks for dark and white variety, respectively.

Bajra (*Pennesetum typhoides*): Like sorghum, this grain is also rich in tannins. Feeding value of bajra is somewhat similar to that of sorghum. CP content is 10-12%. In duck feeding, bajra can be used to some extent in place of maize. ME value is around 2650 Kcal/kg. The inclusion level is 0-25% and 0-45%, for ducklings and adult ducks, respectively.

Tubers

Tapioca Meal (*Manihot esculanta*): Tapioca is cultivated for its root which is normally rich in starch and fructans. Tapioca tubers are mainly used for production of tapioca starch (sabodana) for human consumption. Tapioca is often used in the ration of poultry including duck as an energy source. The tubers are rich in starch but low in protein. Tapioca tuber has 37% DM, 63% moisture, 3.4% CP, 4.3% CF and 27-35% starch. It contains two cyanogenetic glycosides, linamarin and lotaustralin. These are acted upon by enzymes which are usually present in plants and liberate hydrocyanic acid (HCN). However, this can be removed by sun drying or heating. Its inclusion level in ducks is 5-15%

Cereal and Agro-Industrial By-Products

Wheat bran: Coarse outer covering of the wheat kernel is wheat bran. It is bulky in nature. Its palatability is good hence, tasteful but digestibility is low. Wheat bran has 12.5% moisture, 13% in CP, 12% CF and 4.5% fat. In good quality brans, CF content should not contain more than10%. The protein quality of wheat bran is of better quality than that of wheat or maize grain. Wheat bran is rich in niacin and thiamin, but low in riboflavin. Due to presence of good amount CF and pentosans content, wheat bran has laxative in action. Calcium content of wheat bran is low (0.07%) but it is rich in phosphorus (0.35%). It is rich in phytic acid, hence most of the phosphorus is not available to the ducks. Its inclusion level is 10-15% in ducks.

Rice polish: A good quality rice polish has around 12.5% in CP and 13.5% in fat, with a very small amount of CF (2-3%). They are very rich in water soluble vitamins particularly thiamin and niacin. It is very rich in energy. Its ME value is around 3300 Kcal/kg duck ration. The inclusion level of this by-product is 0-40% and 0-50%, in ducklings and adult ducks, respectively. Rice polish may develop rancidity owing to its high fat content. Presence of high amount of unsaturated fatty acid (UFA) is responsible for such rancidity. It is one of the prime feed ingredients for feeding of duck. Inclusion level in case of duck is 10-30%.

Rice bran: Good quality rice bran contains 11-12% CF, 12-14% CP and around 12% of oil with only 0.06% Calcium. However, phosphorus content is more (1.12%). Like rice polish, it also rich in other B-complex vitamins especially, niacin and thiamin. Among the trace elements, it is a rich source of manganese (Mn). It is because of high fat content; rice bran develop rancidity. Nowadays, de-oiled rice bran (DORB) is commonly used in duck rations to avoid the problem of fat rancidity in rice bran. Due to removal of fat, the CP percentage ultimately becomes higher in DORB than rice bran. Rice bran is normally used in the ration of ducks and its inclusion level is 10-20%.

Molasses: It is the by-product of sugar industry. It is rich in soluble carbohydrates but low in protein. However, it is a good source of B-complex vitamin like pantothenic acid, niacin, riboflavin and choline. It can replace 5-10% of cereal grains in a duck ration. It reduces dustiness in feed and improves palatability of the ration. However, it is rich in ash material, potassium. Hence excessive feeding of molasses will lead to lose excreta. Its inclusion level in duck ration is around 5%.

Plant Origin Oil Cakes

Soybean Meal (SBM): Soybean meal is a high protein animal feed ingredient and most commonly used. SBM are generally deoiled type, so oil content is less (0.05-1%). It is an exceptional source for lysine but methionine is the first limiting amino acid. Two grades of SBM are available i.e. 44% CP and 49% CP. SBM is poor source vitamin B-complex and must be provided either as a supplement or in the form of an animal protein such as fish meal. The oil in the soybean has a laxative effect and may result in the production of soft body fat. The ME value is around 2700 Kcal/kg and its inclusion level in both ducklings and adult ducks is 0-40%.

Groundnut Cake (GNC): The CP content of this cake is 45% and it has 10% oil. GNC is an excellent source of arginine but deficient in lysine, methionine and cystine. First limiting amino acid is lysine. GNC is very much prone to attack of fungus Aspergillus. Toxic factor present in it is Aflatoxin, a metabolite of the fungus *Aspergillus flavus*, particularly in warm rainy season. The cake becomes rancid in warm moist climate. Hence, it should not be stored more than 6 weeks in summer or 3-4 months in winter. Ducklings are highly susceptible to aflatoxicosis. According to the process of extraction of oil, the content of oil is variable. ME of GNC is around 2600 Kcal/kg. Inclusion level in both ducklings and duck is 0-40%.

De-oiled Mustard Cake: Oil content is less (1-1.5%) in de-oiled mustard cake. CP content is around 39%. Ca and P content are very much higher (0.29% and 0.39%, respectively). The protein is deficient in lysine. Deoiled type can be used for duck up to 10% of the ration. It has a strong taste and aroma and contains a goitrogenic substance which reduces the growth rate in ducks. Due to feeding of mustard oil cake (have glucosinolates), there is accumulation of fat around heart muscle of duck. Hence, only 10-15% of this cake can be incorporated in duck ration.

Sunflower Meal: Sunflower seed meal is a satisfactory substitute to GNC in starter duck ration and it can replace 100% GNC without any adverse effect on weight gain and feed efficiency. Good quality sunflower meal contains 40-44% protein. The protein is especially rich in methionine (in decorticated variety) and arginine. The first limiting amino acid is lysine. The protein is also low in cystine and glycine also. This cake is safe for ducks for replacement of GNC without any adverse effect on egg production and egg weight. Its ME value is 2230 Kcal/kg and inclusion level in duckling and adult duck is 0-10 and 0-20%, respectively.

Safflower Meal: The CP in decorticated variety of this meal is 40-45%, while in un-decorticated meal it is about 18-20%. Only de-corticated variety is used in duck ration. The meal is low in lysine and methionine. Safflower meal should be used in combination with other lysine rich protein feed ingredients like soybean meal of GNC.

Sesame cake (Til Cake): The quality of protein of this cake is next to GNC. The cake is rich in arginine, leucine, tryptophan and methionine but is relatively low in glycine, cystine and lysine. Feeding of this cake in excessive amount may result in soft body of the duck as the residual oil of the cake is highly unsaturated. The cake is palatable with laxative action. Inclusion level in ducklings is 0-10%, and grower and layers it is 0-20%. CP, CF and EE are 40-50%, 5% and 7%, respectively. Its ME value is 1882 Kcal/kg. Inclusion level in ducklings and duck is 0-10 and 0-20%, respectively.

Animal Origin Protein Sources

Fish Meal: Fish meal provides one of the best quality proteins to ducks. Though, composition of the protein is relatively constant, protein content of various fish meal varies over a range of about 50-75%. It is rich in all essential amino acids, particularly lysine, cystine, methionine and tryptophan. A good quality fishmeal should have at least 50-55% protein, 6.9% oil, 25% minerals, 7.9% Ca and 4.4% P. They are very good source of essential amino acids. Among them it has 4.82% lysine and 1.52% methionine. They are good source of vitamin A, D and B-complex vitamins, particularly choline, patothenic acid, vitamin B_{12} and riboflavin. Fishmeal is the richest source of Vit B_{12}. Its ME value is around 1850 Kcal/kg and inclusion level for both ducklings and adult duck is 0-10%.

Meat and bone Meal: Meat meal is high in protein (45%) and ash (21%). It is an important source of Ca and P (8% and 4%, respectively). The meal is low in trytophan and methionine (first limiting amino acid is tryptophan). It has ME value of 2000 Kcal/kg and inclusion level for both ducklings and adult duck is 0-5%.

Blood Meal: It is an excellent protein source with 80% CP. This meal is one of the richest sources of lysine (6.9% lysine) but its amino acid composition is highly imbalanced. Moreover, it is less palatable and less digestible. It is mainly used to supplement lysine amino acid and hence, its inclusion level for ducks is only 1-2%. The meal is poor in Ca and P (0.33% Ca, 0.26% P). Its ME value is around 2850 Kcal/kg.

Silk Worm Pupae Meal: A good quality silk worm pupae meal will have around 55% CP and 25-27% oil. Therefore, to avoid rancidity problem and to improve keeping quality, de-oiling is advocated. It can replace whole of fishmeal in duck rations. However, replacing 60% fish meal would provide the best results.

Table 1 : Level of inclusion of common Duck feed Ingredients

Feed ingredients	%
Maize	Up to 60
Sorghum	30-40
Bajra	10-20
Wheat	Up to 50
Rice	Up to 40
Rice bran	10-20
De-oiled rice bran	10-20
Rice polish	10-40
Wheat bran	10-15
Tapioca meal	5-15
Molasses	0-5
Maize gluten	0-10
GNC	10-30
Sunflower cake	10-20
Safflower cake	5-15
De-oiled mustard cake	0-5
Soybean meal	Up to 40
Fish meal	5-10
Meat meal	5-10
Blood meal	Up to 3
Silkworm-pupae meal	Up to 6

Table 2 : Chemical composition and Nutritive value of common Poultry/Duck feed ingredients

Ingredients	ME (Kcal/kg)	CP%	CF%	EE%	Ca%	P%	Lysine %	Methionine %
Yellow maize	3340	9	2.2	3.8	0.02	0.28	0.22	0.18
Sorghum white	3200	10	2.3	2.8	0.03	0.28	0.21	0.16
Bajra	2850	11.5	3.5	4.3	0.06	0.33	0.43	0.23
Broken rice	2900	8.5	10.6	1.9	0.08	0.39	0.24	0.16
Wheat	3000	10	2.4	1.8	0.05	0.31	0.30	0.16
Oil	8800	-	-	-	-	-	-	-
DORB	2200	13.5	14	0.6	0.07	1.5	0.6	0.25
Rice polish	3300	12	8	15.1	0.08	1.3	0.5	0.22
Wheat bran	1300	15.7	11	3	0.14	1.15	0.59	0.23
Molasses	2300	3	-	-	1.1	0.12	-	-
Sunflower cake	1900	27	28	1.1	0.37	1	1.13	0.58
SBM	2300	45	6.6	0.8	0.29	0.65	2.7	0.65
GNC-SE	2400	42	13	1	0.2	0.63	1.6	0.45
GNC-EXP	2600	40	13	7.3	0.16	0.56	1.5	0.42
Rapeseed cake	2300	35	11	1.4	0.72	1.12	1.7	0.65
Fish meal	2400	42	1	5	3.73	2.43	3.2	1.1
Meat meal	2400	45	8.7	7.1	8.27	4.1	2.5	0.65
Tapioca	2900	2	9	2	0.1	0.03	0	0

Table 3 : Some common source of Ca and P

Source	Ca (%)	P (%)
Steamed bone meal	29	14
Di-calcium phosphate (DCP)	23	18
Calcium phosphate	17	21
Ground lime stone	38	-
Oyster shell	38	-
Calcium carbonate	40	-
Sodium phosphate	--	22

Steps in duck feed formulation

1. Fixed minor ingredients and slack space (5 kg). This includes nutrient and non-nutrient feed additive and natural feed ingredients added at a later stage to balance the diet.
2. Level the animal protein sources (max. 10 kg). These are added to the diets since they are rich sources of limiting amino acids like lysine, methionine & cystine.

3. The level of cereal by-products is fixed (say, 8 kg).
4. Vegetable protein sources and energy sources are added to provide the required amount of protein (calculation required).
5. Now balance the ME content of the diet. If there is any shortfall then it can be met by supplementation of either animal fat or vegetable oil or maize grain depending on the availability and cost.
6. Balance the P content of the diet: Here available P is considered.
7. Balance the Ca content. If there is a shortfall then it can be met by supplementation of lime stone, bone meal, etc.
8. Maximum supplementation for salt is 0.3% (ICAR, 2013). But, when fish meal, meat meals are used then 0.2% supplementation is required.
9. Balance the limiting amino acids in the diet. Animal protein sources are rich sources for lysine and methionine. Among vegetable sources, soybean meal is a rich source of lysine. They are also available in synthetic form.
10. Balance the CF content of the diet.

Feed Additives in Duck Rations

Probiotics: These are live microbes which act as feed supplements having beneficial effect on the host animal by improving its intestinal microbial balance. Growth as well as production performance of the duck is improved due to the use of probiotics. *Lactobacillus acidophilus, Aspergillus oryzae, Saccharomyces cerevisiae* etc. microorganisms which act as as probiotics.

Prebiotics: Fructo-Oligosaccharides (FOS) and Mannan-Oligosaccharides (MOS) are the common examples of prebiotics. They improve health, growth and laying performance. The attachment of pathogenic harmful bacteria to the intestine is inhibited by the prebiotics, thereby preventing colonization and disease. Probiotic microorganisms are also get benefitted due to proliferation of the beneficial (probiotic) bacteria which ultimately inhibit the growth of more harmful bacteria.

Antibiotics: Antibiotics are generally used in small doses in the ration to prevent microbial infections. It shows better result in ducks which are given to all vegetable protein diets than those getting animal protein diets. Moreover, Antibiotic shows better result in an unhygienic condition than when used in hygienic condition. The growth rate may vary between 10-20% and reducing the feed intake by about 2-5%. The efficiency of feed utilization is improved by 5-8%. The dose rate of antibiotic is normally 5-15mg/ kg feed. e.g. Flavomycin, Virginamycin, Bacitracin, etc.

Antioxidants: Fats are prone to oxidation. So, rancidity develops in fat which reduces palatability of the ration with digestive upsets. The antioxidants mop up the free radicals. So, fat and fat soluble vitamins are stabilized. Antioxidants are available in two forms i.e. natural and synthetic. Vitamin E and vitamin C are natural antioxidant while DPPD (diphenyl-paraphenylene-diamine), BHA (Butylated hydroxyl anisole), BHT (Butylated hydroxyl toluene) and Ethoxyquin are the most common synthetic antioxidants.

Mycotoxin binder: Mycotoxins are produced from various fungus which are harmful to ducks. *Aspergillus, Fusarium, Penicellium* are the name of some important fungus. Important mycotoxins are aflatoxins, zearalenone, ochratoxin A, etc. Mineral clays like aluminosilicates (Hydrated sodium calcium aluminosilicate i.e. HSCAS) are commonly used in duck feeds as toxin binders.

Enzymes: Enzymes as feed additives, improves the digestibility of certain feedstuffs. Maize and soyabean meal are the most commonly used feed ingredients for poultry including ducks. High cost of these ingredients has compelled the feed manufacturers to include feed stuffs like wheat, oats, barley, sunflower seed meal, rapeseed meal, etc while formulating ration for poultry/ duck. However, the digestibility of these ingredients is not satisfactory. The non-starch polysaccharides (NSPs) present in the cereal grains are cellulose, arabinoxylans and betaglucans. Hence, commercial enzymes like xylanase, arabinase, mannase, glucanase, pectinase, cellulase, phytase etc. are being used in the duck ration.

Energy requirements of starter, grower and layer ducks

Ducks eat primarily for fulfilling the energy requirement. Once its energy requirement is fulfilled then it will not take food temporarily. So, ducks eat for calories which mean their energy intake is maintained at constant level. The energy requirement of duck is specified usually in terms of kilocalories ME per kg of the diet. The feed consumption of ducks is inversely related to the dietary energy level. Ducks takes more of a low energy diet than of a high energy diet. Ducks if kept on a high energy diet then carcass fat will also be higher. If ducklings are kept on low energy diet, then a decreased growth rate would be noted.

Feeding of layer ducks

Nutrient requirement and feeding of starter ducklings

During the embryonic development only half of the ME present in the egg is utilized. Rest half of the ME will be utilized by the hatched ducklings within

60-72 hours. This energy is adequate to maintain the body temperature of ducklings for 60-72 hours. Some recommended no feed should be offered to the ducklings during this period, otherwise there will be delay in absorption of the yolk. Higher mortality has also been observed in ducklings when feed is provided immediately after hatching. But now-a-days it is recommended that first feed should be fed as soon as possible and there is no need to wait for absorption of yolk. Ducklings normally do not consume much of feed during the first few days but will at least be able to locate the feeders. Hence, it is advisable to feed to ducklings as soon as possible after hatching.

The ducklings immediately after their hatching are reared in the brooding house for four weeks. Duck starter ration should be provided to ducklings during this time. A duck starter diet containing 20.5% CP, 1% lysine, 0.45% methionine and 2800 kcal ME/kg diet should be provided to the newly hatched duckling. The feed should have 1% Ca and 0.42% available P with all trace minerals and vitamins. The ratio of desirable calcium and available P should be 2.38:1in the starter ration. As the ducklings always suffer from riboflavin and niacin deficiency hence, adequate riboflavin and niacin should be in the starter feed. On a riboflavin deficient diet, there is retardation of growth in ducklings after 2 or 3 days and frequently die within 4-7 days. In niacin deficiency, ducklings suffer from bowed leg condition. The leg becomes very weak and such leg weakness results in complete crippling. Common salt should not be more than 0.30%. Watery droppings and wet litter condition is a very common condition in a high salt ration. The mash feed should be made moistened with water. The ducklings must get fresh drinking water round the clock.

General idea to formulate a starter ration

Cereals or grains/ (maize/wheat, tapioca and combination of these): 50-60%

Cereal by-products (rice bran/wheat bran or combination of these): 5-10%

Vegetable origin proteins (GNC cake/soybean meal/til cake or combination of these): 20-22%

Animal origin protein source (fish meal/meat meat/silk worm meal): 8%

Common salt: 0.3%

Di-Calcium Phosphate: 1.5%

Limestone powder: 1%

Trace minerals: 0.1%

Vitamin AB_2D_3: 0.02%

Nutrient requirement and feeding of grower/rearer ducks

Grower/rearer feed should be provided to the growing ducks from 8 weeks and is continued up to 18 to 20 weeks period. The grower ducks should be fed with a rearer diet containing a minimum of 15% CP, 0.6 to 0.75% lysine, 0.3-35% methionine and 2500 kcal ME/kg diet. The feed should have all trace minerals and vitamins including 1% Ca and 0.35% available P. The ratio of desirable Ca and available P should be 2.85:1in the layer ration.

A proper body weight must be maintained by the grower ducks prior to their laying. Hence, restricted feeding is practiced in the grower ducks. It is done between 12-20 weeks (3-5 months). Excess feeding during grower phase leads to obesity. The obesity severely affects the reproductive performance of ducks and limits the numbers of eggs laid and the fertility of those eggs. Restricted feeding is also practiced in young grower ducks to delay onset of sexual maturity, so that egg size can be improved and uniform sized eggs can be got from a flock. Here, nutrient intake is reduced below the normal level. Restricted feeding may result in lower feed cost per dozen egg produced. Delayed sexual maturity helps in getting larger eggs even during the initial phase of production and more number of eggs in a particular season.

Effects of feed restriction of grower birds

1. Due to restriction of feed, feed consumed by the growers is less. So, feed costs are reduced a lot.
2. Total feed conversion efficiency for egg production is better in controlled feed group ducks than the ducks of full-fed group in grower phase.
3. Restricted feed fed group birds reach a higher peak of egg production as compared to those fed as free choice during grower phase.
4. After the sexual maturity, restricted feed fed group ducks show a higher average rate of egg production compared to those fed as free choice during grower phase.

Methods of restricted feeding: Feeding of low energy diet by diluting the feed with fibrous material of low nutrient density may be provided to the ducks. But it increases rearing cost. In other method, quantitative feed restriction may be practiced where 85-90% of normal intake that is consumed by a similar duck on an *ad libitum* basis, offered daily. This type of feed restriction may be continued from 9th week to 20th week of age. A low protein, low lysine diet will bring delayed maturity. A diet containing 14-15% protein is used. Such diets are actually low lysine diets since low lysine grains form the bulk. It is reported that low protein and low lysine diet are able to delay the sexual maturity than the quantitative feed restriction.

General idea to formulate a grower duck ration

Cereals or grains and tubers (maize/wheat, tapioca and combination of these): 50-60%

Cereal byproducts (rice bran/wheat bran or combination of these): 15-20%

Vegetable origin proteins (GNC/soybean meal/til cake or combination of these): 12-14%

Animal origin protein (fish meal/meat meat/silk worm meal or their combination): 5%

Common salt: 0.3%

Di-Calcium Phosphate: 1.5%

Limestone powder: 1%

Trace minerals: 0.1%

Nutrient requirement and feeding of layer ducks

From 20-22 week onwards, a layer diet containing a minimum of 16.5-18% CP, 0.75% lysine, 0.30% methionine, 2650 kcal ME/kg diet, 3% calcium and 0.35% available P with all trace minerals and vitamins should be provided and it should continue during the entire laying period. The ratio of desirable Ca and available P should be 8.5:1in the layer ration. Around 5-6% oyster shell (38% Ca) or limestone powder (38% Ca) is to be added in a layer ration in order to get the desired level of Ca% in the layer ration. Enough Ca is required in the diet of duck for formation of eggs and also for the high-quality egg shells. High egg shell quality is required for prevention of breakage during handling and for hatchability. The requirement of Ca is especially high because calcium carbonate makes up approximately 98% of the shell. Egg shell contains 2.2 g of Ca and only 50-60% of the dietary Ca is absorbed, then approx. 4g of dietary Ca is required for each egg. The average daily feed requirement for a layer duck is 150-175g. Restriction of feed to some extent during the laying period is found beneficial.

General idea to formulate a layer duck ration

Cereals or grains and tubers (maize/wheat, tapioca and combination of these): 50-55%

Cereal byproducts (rice bran/wheat bran or combination of these): 10%

Vegetable origin proteins (GNC/soybean meal/til cake or combination of these): 18%

Animal origin proteins (fish meal/meat meat/silk worm meal): 8%

Common salt: 0.3%

Di-Calcium Phosphate: 1.5%

Oyester shell/ Limestone powder: 6.5%

Trace minerals: 0.1%

Effect of diet on duck egg production and egg hatchability

Deficiency of Ca, Mn, protein, vitamin A, vitamin D, vitamin B_2 and Choline causes a reduction in egg production or even cessation of egg production.

- ***Vitamins***: Amount of vitamins present in the egg depends upon concentration of vitamins present in the breeder diet which in turn influences the hatchability of egg and viability of ducklings. Vitamin A, D, E, K, Riboflavin, Thiamin, Pantothenic acid, Nicotinic acid, Pyridoxine, Folic acid, Biotin and Cyanocobalamine are essential for normal development of embryo and hatchability. Deficiency of vitamin D_3 also causes reduction in hatchability. During embryonic development most of the vit. D_3 is utilized by the growing embryo and hence no significant storage of vit D_3 is found in ducklings.
- ***Minerals***: Minerals required for normal hatchability: Ca, P, Mn, Zn, Mg, Fe, Cu, I, Mn and Se. Both deficiency and excess of dietary Ca causes reduced hatchability. Mn is required for formation of strong egg shell and good hatchability. Deficiency of Mn causes abnormal embryonic development and heavy mortality. Excess Se has also adverse effect on egg hatchability. Deficiency of iron causes reduced hatchability of egg. Deficiency of iodine causes delayed hatching, poor hatchability yolk retention in ducklings.
- ***Energy***: High energy intake leads to slight increase in egg yolk weight due to synthesis of body fat and yolk lipoproteins. Now, if protein, vitamins and minerals proportion is not increased in the same manner then a general or specific deficiency may develop and causes reduced hatchability.
- ***Protein and amino acids***: Marginal deficiency of protein causes a reduction in the egg size. As the amino acid composition remains unaltered, a smaller size egg is laid. If dietary protein level is increased beyond 15% then hatchability of eggs does not increase. However, if dietary protein level is decreased below 12% then hatchability of eggs reduces drastically.
- ***Fat and essential fatty acid:*** Amount of lenoleic acid present in the egg yolk depends upon concentration of this fatty acid present in the breeder diet which in turn influences the hatchability of egg and viability of ducklings. Lenoleic acid is essential in breeder duck for normal hatchability. Severe deficiency of lenoleic acid may lead to 0% hatchability.

Drinking water

Duck needs plenty of clean and safe drinking water round the clock. Water sanitizer may be used at least 30 minutes before drinking to reduce the pathogen load in water. Water requirements increase exponentially as the temperature rises; as temperatures approach 32°C, water requirement increases dramatically. Therefore, during hot weathers, when evening temperature is above 32°C then drinking water must be provided till the temperature of the shed decreased to 26.5°C.

Table 4 : Suggested Nutrient requirements for Duck recommended by the ICAR' 2013

Characteristic	**Starter Duck (0-8 wks)**	**Grower Duck (8-16 wks)**	**Rearer Duck (16-20 wks)**	**Layer Duck (20 wks onward)**
Moisture, % (Max.)	11.00	11.00	11.00	11.00
CP, % (Min.)	**20.50**	**16.50**	**15.00**	**16.50**
CF, % (Max.)	7.00	8.00	8.00	6.00
Acid insoluble ash, % (Max.)	4.00	4.00	4.00	3.00
Salt, % (Max.)	0.30	0.30	0.30	0.30
Calcium, % (Min.)	1.00	1.00	1.00	3.00
Phosphorous (Available), % (Min.)	0.42	0.35	0.35	0.35
Linoleic Acid, % (Min.)	1.00	1.00	0.08	1.00
Lysine, % (Min.)	1.00	0.75	0.60	0.75
Methionine, % (Min.)	0.45	0.35	0.30	0.30
Methionine + cystine, %	0.85	0.65	0.60	0.75
Metabolizable Energy (Kcal/ Kg) Min.	**2800**	**2650**	**2500**	**2650**
Minerals and Vitamins:				
Sodium	0.17	0.15	0.15	0.17
Chlorine	0.12	0.12	0.12	0.12
Manganese, mg/kg	60.00	50.00	40.00	50.00
Vitamin A, IU/Kg	3200	2250	2250	4000
Vitamin D_3 , IU/Kg	400	350	350	650
Riboflavin, mg/kg	5.00	4.00	4.00	6.00
Pantothenic acid, mg/kg	10.00	8.00	8.00	12.00
Nicotinic Acid, mg/kg	60.00	55.00	50.00	50.00
Biotin, mg/kg	0.10	0.10	0.10	0.10
Folic Acid, mg/kg	0.60	0.40	0.40	0.60
Choline, mg/kg	1000	750	500	750
Vitamin E, mg/kg	20.00	20.00	15.00	20.00
Vitamin K, mg/kg	2.5	2.00	2.00	2.5
Pyridoxine, mg/kg	3.00	2.50	2.50	3.00

Table 5 : Suggested Nutrient requirements for egg and meat type duck used at CPDO, Hessarghata.

Characteristic	**Starter Duck**	**Grower Duck**	**Layer Duck**	**Broiler (Vigova-M) Starter Duck**	**Broiler (Vigova-M) Finisher Duck**
Moisture, % (Max.)	11.00	11.00	11.00	11.00	11.00
CP, % (Min.)	20.00	16.00	18.00	23.00	20.00
CF, % (Max.)	7.00	8.00	8.00	6.00	6.00
Acid insoluble ash, % (Max.)	4.00	4.00	4.00	3.00	3.00
Salt, % (Max.)					
Calcium, % (Min.)	0.60	0.60	0.60	0.60	0.60
Phosphorous (Available), %	1.00	1.00	3.00	1.20	1.20
(Min.)	0.50	0.50	0.50	0.50	0.50
Linoleic Acid, % (Min.)					
Lysine, % (Min.)	1.00	1.00	1.00	1.00	1.00
Methionine, % (Min.)	0.90	0.60	0.65	1.20	1.00
Methionine + cystine, %	0.30	0.25	0.30	0.50	0.35
Metabolizable Energy (Kcal/Kg)	0.60	0.50	0.55	0.90	0.70
Min.	2600	2500	2600	2800	2900
Minerals and Vitamins:					
Manganese, mg/kg	90.00	50.00	55.00	90.00	90.00
Iodine, mg/kg	1.00	1.00	1.00	1.00	1.00
Iron, mg/kg	120.00	90.00	75.00	120.00	120.00
Zinc, mg/kg	60.00	50.00	75.00	60.00	60.00
Copper, mg/kg	12.00	9.00	9.00	12.00	120.00
Vitamin A, IU/Kg	6000	6000	6000	6000	6000
Vitamin D_3, IU/Kg	600	600	1200	600	600
Thiamin, mg/kg	5.00	3.00	3.00	5.00	5.00
Riboflavin, mg/kg	6.00	5.00	5.00	6.00	6.00
Pantothenic acid, mg/kg	15.00	15.00	15.00	15.00	15.00
Nicotinic Acid, mg/kg	70.00	60.00	60.00	70.00	70.00
Biotin, mg/kg	0.20	0.15	0.15	0.20	0.20
Vitamin B_{12}, mg/kg	0.015	0.010	0.010	0.015	0.015
Folic Acid, mg/kg	1.00	0.50	0.50	1.00	1.00
Choline, mg/kg	1300	900	800	1400	1000
Vitamin E, mg/kg	15.00	10.00	10.00	15.00	15.00
Vitamin k, mg/kg	1.00	1.00	1.00	1.00	1.00
Pyridoxine, mg/kg	5.00	5.00	5.00	5.00	5.00

Mineral mixture per 100 kg diet: Ferrous sulphate: 20 g; Manganese sulphate, 50 g; Zinc sulphate, 25 g; Copper sulphate, 1.5 g and Potassium iodate, 100 mg.

Vitamin mixture per 100 kg diet: Vit A, 800,000 IU; Vit. D_3, 1, 00,000 ICU; Riboflavin, 400 mg; folic acid, 100 mg and Niacin 5g

Feeding schedule of Pekin Ducks

The Pekin ducks are the most popular meat type duck for table purpose in the world. White Pekin ducks are of broiler type. In 8 weeks of rearing their body weight become 3.3-3.6 kg with a feed consumption of 9.6-9.9 kg. It is fast growing and has low feed consumption with fine quality of meat. It attains about 2.2 to 2.5 kgs of body weight in 42 days of age, with a feed conversion ratio of 1:2.3 to 2.7 kgs.

Table 6 : Approximate body weights and feed consumption of white pekin ducks (male) up to 8 weeks of age

Age (weeks)	**Body wt. (g)**	**Avg. daily intake(g)**	**Weekly avg. Feed intake (g)**	**Cumulative feed intake (kg)**
0	60 (initial wt.)	-	-	-
1	270	30	210	210
2	780	110	770	980
3	1380	160	1120	2100
4	1960	185	1295	3395
5	2490	200	1400	4795
6	2960	230	1610	6405
7	3340	240	1680	8085
8	3610	240	1680	9765

Table 7 : Nutrient requirements of white Pekin ducks as percentages or units per kilogram of diet (90 percent dry matter)

Nutrients **ME Kcal/kg**	**Unit**	**0-2 Weeks** **2,900**	**2-7 Weeks** **3,000**	**Breeding** **2,900**
Protein	**%**	**22**	**16**	**15**
Arginine	%	1.1	1.0	1.0
Isoleucine	%	0.63	0.46	0.38
Leucine	%	1.26	0.91	0.76
Lysine	**%**	**0.90**	**0.65**	**0.60**
Methionine	**%**	**0.40**	**0.30**	**0.27**
Methionine + cystine	%	0.70	0.55	0.50
Tryptophan	%	0.23	0.17	0.14
Valine	%	0.78	0.56	0.47
Macro-minerals				
Calcium	**%**	**0.65**	**0.60**	**2.75**
Chloride	%	0.12	0.12	0.12
Magnesium	mg	500	500	500
Nonphytate phosphorus	%	0.40	0.30	0.30

Sodium	%	0.15	0.15	0.15
Trace minerals				
Manganese	mg	50	-	-
Selenium	mg	0.20	-	-
Zinc	mg	60	-	-
Fat soluble vitamins				
A	**IU**	**2,500**	**2,500**	**4,000**
D_3	**IU**	**400**	**400**	**900**
E	IU	10	10	10
K	mg	0.5	0.5	0.5
Water soluble vitamins				
Niacin	mg	55	55	55
Pantothenic acid	mg	11.0	11.0	11.0
Pyridoxine	mg	2.5	2.5	3.0
Riboflavin	mg	4.0	4.0	4.0

Table 8 : Feed formulae for Ducks followed at C.P.D.O. , Hessarghata

Ingredient (%)	**Khaki Campbell Duck**			**White Broilder Duck**		
	Starter	**Grower**	**Layer**	**Starter**	**Grower**	**Layer**
Wheat	45	48	42	60	40	40
Yellow Maize	-	-	10	-	29	20
D.O.R.B.	14	25.5	6.5	-	10	-
Soyabeam Meal	25	15	20	25	10	20
Fish Meal	10	6	10	10	6	10
Lucern leaf meal	2	2	2	2	2	2
Mineral mixture	2.5	2.5	2.5	2.5	2.5	2.5
Shell grit	-	-	5.5	-	-	5
D.C.P.	1.0	0.5	1.0	-	-	-
Vitamin mixture	0.5	0.5	0.5	0.5	0.5	0.5
Total	**100.0**	**100.0**	**100.0**	**100.0**	**100.0**	**100.0**
Vitamin mixture in g (per 100 kg)						
Vitamin AB_2D_3 K	25	25	30	25	25	30
Vitamin B+E	25	25	30	25	25	30
Niacinamide	5	5	5	5	5	5
Choline chloride	50	50	50	50	50	50
Antibiotic	50	50	50	50	50	50
A.P.F. – 100	20	20	20	20	20	20
U.T.T.P.	20	20	20	20	20	20
Total	**195g**	**195g**	**205g**	**195g**	**195g**	**205g**

Table 9 : Feed scale for Khaki Campbell Duck

Age (Weeks)	Feed consumption/ bird/week/kg.	Age (Weeks)	Feed consumption/ bird/week/kg.
1	0.115	13	0.595
2	0.255	14	0.605
3	0.425	15	0.630
4	0.620	16	0.705
Total	**1.415**	**Total**	**2.535**
5	0.720	**Progressive total**	**9.945**
6	0.770	17	0.615
7	0.785	18	0.655
8	0.790	19	0.665
Total	**3.065**	20	0.745
Progressive Total	**4.480**	**Total**	**2.680**
9	0.690	**Progressive Total**	**12.625**
10	0.730	21	0.775
11	0.755	22	0.945
12	0.755	23	0.950
Total	**2.930**	24	0.955
Progressive Total	**7.410**	**Total**	**3.625**
		Progressive Total	**16.250**

Table 10 : Computation of Duck rations (composition of duck rations for three different phases)

Ingredients	Duck starter (%)	Duck grower (%)	Duck layer (%)
Maize/broken wheat	54.3	60.3	57.3
Wheat Bran	14	19	9
Soybean meal	19.5	10.5	18
Dry fish	10	8	8
Bone meal	1	1	1
Mineral mixture	1	1	1
Oyster shell	-	-	5.5
Salt	0.2	0.2	0.2
Toxin binder	0.08	0.08	0.08
Antibiotics/100kg	20g	20g	20g
Vitamin AB_2D_3 /100kg	20g	20g	20g

N. B. As maize has been used instead of wheat; the level of mycotoxin binder has been increased accordingly (from normal 0.05% to 0.08%).

Table 11 : Daily feed intake and gain in body weight of Khaki Campbell Duck

Mash/ Pellet	**Age (Weeks)**	**Avg. daily feed intake/ duck (g)**	**Total feed intake/duck/ week(g)**	**Live weight/ duck (g)**	**Progressive feed intake**
Duck starter (0-8 weeks)					
	0 day	-	A little	30 g	
	1st week	15	105	80g	
	2	35	245	120g	
	3	60	420	250g	
	4	90	630	350g	
		Total	1400 gram		1400 gram
	5	105	735		
	6	110	770		
	7	115	805		
	8	115	805		
		Total	3115 gram		4515 gram
Duck grower (9-20 weeks)					
	9	100	700		
	10	105	735		
	11	110	770		
	12	110	770		7490 gram
	13	85	595		
	14	90	630		
	15	90	630		
	16	100	700		10045 gram
	17	90	630		
	18	95	665		
	19	95	665		
	20	105	735	2000g	12740 gram
		Total	8225 gram		
Duck layer (21st week onwards)					
	21	110	770		
	22	135	945		
	23	135	945		
	24	140	980		16380 gram
		Total	3640 gram		

Table 12 : Performance chart of Khaki Campbell (egg type)

1	Age at first egg	120 days
2	Age at 50% production	146 days
3	Annual Egg Production	250 eggs
4	Egg weight at 40 weeks	66 g
5	Body weight at 40 weeks	1.80 kg
6	Daily feed consumption per bird	120 – 130 g
7	Ducklings mortality (0-8 weeks)	2 – 3%
8	Grower mortality (8 – 20 weeks)	0.2 – 0.5%
9	Adult mortality (20 – 72 weeks)	5 – 7%

Table 13 : Performance chart of Vigova Super-M (meat type)

1	Day old body weight	47 – 48 g
2	Body weight at 4 weeks	1.3 – 1.5 kg
3	Feed consumption up to 4 weeks	3.0 – 3.2 kg
4	Body weight at 6 weeks	2.3 – 2.5 kg
5	Feed consumption up to 6 weeks	5.8 – 6.2 kg
6	Mortality (0-6 weeks)	2 – 3%

Table 14 : Average body weight and feed consumption of broiler ducks at 6 weeks of age

Age (Weeks)	**Body Weight (kg)**	**Daily feed intake (g)**	**Feed Consumption**	
			Weekly (kgs.)	**Cumulative (kgs.)**
1.	0.183	20	0.140	0.140
2.	0.526	80	0.560	0.700
3.	1.048	144	1.008	1.708
4.	1.533	180	1.260	2.968
5.	2.082	203	1.421	4.389
6.	2.498	200	1.400	5.789

Table 15 : Daily feed intake of Vigova Super–M broiler duck in Regional Exotic Duck Breeding Farm, Tripura

Day	**Feed intake (g)**
1st week	96g/week i.e 13.7 g/day/duckling
2nd week	331g/week i.e. 47.2g/day/duckling
3rd week	580g/week i.e 82g/day/duck
4th week	754g/week i.e. 107g/day/duck
29 to 120 days	150-200 gm/day
Adult (120 days and above)	190-240gm/day

Aflatoxicosis

Aflatoxicosis is a disease condition caused by mycotoxins (aflatoxins) produced by the mold *Aspergillus flavus*. Feedstuffs like groundnut, maize, sorghum, rice polish, cottonseed cake and other tropical feeds are highly susceptible to this mold infestation. Mold growth gets a favorable atmosphere due to improper drying of grains, rain and humid weather. Though ducks are the most susceptible to aflatoxins, the ducklings are more susceptible than the adult ducks. Among the same species, the ducklings of Khaki Campbell are the most susceptible to aflatoxin followed by Minikos and White Pekins ducklings. Ducks are about 200 times more sensitive than broiler and layer birds. Chickens can tolerate to the extent of 0.20 ppm, whereas, in ducks it is just 0.03 ppm. The molds themselves are not intrinsically toxigenic but the metabolites that are liberated on the feedstuffs are very much toxic. Their favourable condition to grow and colonize themselves in aerobic conditions with moisture content of feedstuffs over and above 15% with an optimum temperature of 24- 25^{0}C. B_1, B_2, and G_1 and G_2 are the four major aflatoxins. Among them the most important toxin is B_1 aflatoxin because of its toxicity and concentration in moldy feeds is maximum. Presence of a very high level of enzyme in the liver of ducklings to convert aflatoxin B_1 to "Aflatoxicol" is mainly responsible for toxicity of aflatoxin B_1.

It is always suggested to keep away from moldy feeds in order to control the infestation. Particularly during and after monsoon season, there should have a periodical checkup of feed ingredients and finished feed for aflatoxin. Highly vulnerable feedstuffs like maize, GNC etc. should be avoided during formulation of duck ration. Maize can be replaced by rice, wheat or other similar grains while GNC can be replaced by other plant origin proteins like soybean meal, til cake etc. Hydrated sodium calcium alumino silicate (HSCAS) may be used as mycotoxin binder @ 0.5-1% of the ration of duck.

Methyl-mercury and duck: Sometimes mercury is found to be deposited in the soil beds of river, ponds, lakes or any other natural bodies. This may take place due to the effluents of industrial wastes having high concentration of mercury. This inorganic mercury is converted to methyl-mercury by the microorganisms present in the soil bed. In fact, they methylate the mercury to form this fat-soluble compound (methyl-mercury). The methyl mercury is taken up by the algae and other aquatic plans which in turn is taken up by the small fishes. The ducks reared in extensive system consume these affected aquatic plants and small fishes and methyl-mercury is deposited in the fatty tissues and mainly in liver. Humans may be affected with mercury poisoning on consuming such affected meat and eggs of duck for a long period.

References

Ash, W.J., 1976. "Raising ducks", U.S.D.A., Farmer Bulletin No. 2215.

Banerjee G.C. Poultry. Third Edition. Oxford and IBH Publishing.

Dean, W.F., 1986. Nutrition of the Pekin Duck in North America: An Update. Proc. 1986 Cornell Nutrition Conference, Ithaca, N.Y., pp.44-51.

Elkin, R.G., 1987. A review of duck nutrition research. World's Poultry Science 43, No. 2:84-106.

Farrell, D.J., and P. Stapleton, eds. 1986. Duck Production Science and World Practice. Printed by the University of New England, Armidale.

http://www.cpdosrbng.kar.nic.in

Indian Council of Agricultural Research, 2013, Nutrient requirements of duck.

Mullin, J. 1987. Game Bird Propagation – Wildlife Harvest System. Arrowhead Hunting & Conservation Club, Goose Lake, Iowa 52750.

National Research Council, 1994. Nutrient requirements of poultry. National Academy Press, Washington.

Reddy D. V. Applied Nutrition (Livestock, Poultry, Rabbit and Laboratory Animals). Third Edition. Oxford and IBH Publishing.

S.K. Ranjan. Animal Nutrition in Tropics: Fourth Revised edition. Vikas Publishing House Pvt. Ltd.

6

Non-Infectious Diseases of Duck

Poultry in general and duck in particular are not free from diseases though they are far more cold-hardy and healthier than the chickens. Infectious agents are not the only cause of diseases in poultry. However, it can be affected by a wide range of diseases that is caused by the non-infectious agents and it can range from cases of cannibalism to various nutritional related diseases or disorders. Unlike the infectious diseases which tends to affect a whole litter, non-infectious diseases may however be sometime confined to a single bird.

Non infectious diseases can be basically categorized into subgroups like –

a. Nutritional disorders
b. Toxins and poisoning in ducks
c. Miscellaneous disorders

Nutritional Disorders

Nutrients like amino acids, vitamins, inorganic chemical elements, carbohydrates, fats, energy, water and oxygen are essential for the normal development and growth, livability, work and reproduction of the animals. Proper concentration and balance of these nutrients is required to be effective. There is an established nutrient requirement for the growing chicks and poults, as well as for laying –type hens and for broiler and turkey breeders.

The occurrence of nutritional disorders in birds are due to multiple factors some of which are human errors such as the omission of one ingredient or two or groups of vitamins, improper mixing of the diet constituents, improper storage or storage facility, miscomputations in feed formulations and misfeeding to wrong species or sex or age of the birds. Some other important factors that influence the nutritional diseases include poor nutritive value of an ingredient, nutrient and mineral interactions, poor shelf life and insufficient feed availability. Besides, the above-mentioned factors, sometimes due to the poor health condition of the birds caused by the infectious agents it also results in inappetence, poor feed intake, dysphagia, maldigestion, malabsorption, decreased storage or utilization, increased excretion or secretion and increased requirements that can also cause the disorders.

Vitamin Deficiencies in Duck

A vitamin deficiency causes multiple signs in poultry arises due to the inadvertent omission of a complete vitamin premix from the birds' diet. In general, signs of B vitamin deficiencies appear first as there is no storage of water-soluble vitamins in body. Besides, fat-soluble vitamins are stored in the body, hence it often takes longer for these deficiencies to affect the bird and it may take months for vitamin A deficiency to affect adult birds.

Problems with water soluble vitamins such as B are soon observed because they are not stored to any extent, even excreted via the urine if in excess, while fat soluble vitamin deficiencies can take longer to develop because of adipose tissue and liver storage in older birds. The common practice in poultry farming to include vitamins and minerals in feed composite premixes which leads to the less like hood occurrence of individual classical vitamin deficiencies, unless one has been omitted from a premix. It is therefore not unusual to see a situation where the entire premix has been inadvertently excluded with as a consequence, the development of a complex array of clinical signs.

Treatment and prevention rely on an adequate dietary supply, usually microencapsulated gelatin or starch along with an antioxidant. Vitamin destruction in feeds is a factor of time, temperature, and humidity. For most feeds, efficacy of vitamins is little affected over 2-months storage within mixed feed. Problems with water soluble vitamins such as B complex are soon observed because they are not stored to any extent, even excreted via the urine if in excess, while fat soluble vitamin deficiencies can take longer to develop because of adipose tissue and liver storage in older birds.

Vitamin A Deficiency (Hypovitaminosis A)

Vitamin A is an essential fat-soluble vitamin and is predominantly stored in the liver. Vitamin A comes from two sources: one from animal source i.e retinoids and includes retinol and the other from the plant source called the carotenoids and it includes the beta-carotene.

Vitamin A is essential for carrying out the various body functions. The most important ones being the embryonic development, formation of the organ, functioning of the normal immune systems, maintenance of the integrity of the mucous membranes, skin and growth of bones, development of the eye and vision, regulating and maintaining the stability of cell membranes and nerve sheaths, synthesis of adrenal cortical hormones (corticosterone), regulation of thyroxin output and production of the red blood cells.

Vitamin supplements are almost universally used in most of the poultry diets, the likelihood of deficiency is very rare in the present context.

Predisposing factors for Vitamin A deficiency in duck-

- Starved or the malnourished chronic sick ducks.
- Feeding feeds which have been stored for a longer duration of time above 2 months.
- Minimal access to the fresh forages.
- Post-coccidial infection as it leads to damage of the microvilli of the intestinal wall and also causes the destruction of vitamin A in the gut.
- Parasitic load in the GIT (roundworms, tapeworms, flukes)
- Imbalanced vitamin supplementation in the diet.
- Increased susceptibility to infections, especially bumblefoot and aspergillosis in the event of vitamin A deficiency.

Clinical signs

- Development of white plaques on the roof of the mouth or base of the tongue due to the erosion of the mucus membrane of the oral cavity and sinus.
- Defects in growth and differentiation of epithelial tissues, frequently resulting in keratinization. Loss in the function of the alimentary, genital, reproductive, respiratory and urinary tracts.

Stunted growth

- Oral lesions (white plaques)
- Weakness
- Swelling of eyelids
- Egg production drops markedly, hatchability decreases, and embryonic mortality increases
- Development of pustules in the mucous membrane of the esophagus that usually affect the respiratory tract and also paralysis in young ones.
- Conjunctivitis
- Incoordination (ataxia)
- Sinusitis and poor ruffled feathers.

Diagnosis

- History
- Clinical signs
- Physical examination and
- Analysis of the fed content

Line of treatment

- Supplementation of Vitamin A in the diet 2 times at normally recommended level, should be fed for 2 weeks. Vitamin A can be administered through the drinking water.

The dietary requirement of vitamin A in the diet of ducks is as follows

0 to 7 weeks 8,000 IU

7 to 20 weeks 5,000 IU

8 Older than 20 weeks 10,000 IU

Vitamin A requirements are higher under stressful conditions such as extremely hot weather, viral infections, and altered thyroid function.

Prevention

- Provision of a proper balanced diet with fresh greens.
- Discard the duck feed that is suspected to be stale and kept for a long duration in the store.

Vitamin D_3 Deficiency

Vitamin D is a fat-soluble vitamin that regulates the calcium homeostasis and is required for the normal absorption and metabolism of calcium and phosphorus and is vital for the bone health.

Vitamin D is present in two forms- Ergocalciferol (Vitamin D_2) and Chole-calciferol (Vitamin D_3). Vitamin D is normally produced by ultraviolet (UV) light acting on 7-dehydrocholesterol in the skin and it can also be absorbed from the feed. A deficiency can result in rickets in young growing chickens or in osteoporosis and/or poor eggshell quality in laying hens, even though the diet may be well supplied with calcium and phosphorus. Like vitamins A and E, unless vitamin D3 is stabilized, it is destroyed by oxidation, which is increased by heat, moisture and trace minerals. Vitamin D3 is absorbed from the intestinal tract in association with fats as it is fat-soluble vitamins. Like the others, it requires the presence of the bile salts for absorption.

Clinical Signs

- In laying ducks due to absence or deficiency of vitamin D in a duck's diet, the absorption of the calcium gets affected, resulting in calcium deficiency which ultimately leads to a drop in egg production or abnormal egg shells.
- Development of hypocalcaemia or rickets, resulting in stunted growth in growing ducklings with inadequate levels of vitamin D.

- Development of cardiovascular disease, skin conditions, cancer, and autoimmune disorders in vitamin D deficiency.
- Decrease in egg production with poor egg shell quality
- Thin egg shells
- Stunted growth
- Rickets or hypocalcaemia in young growing ducks
- Beaks and claws become soft and pliable
- Abnormal blackening of feathers
- Soft, spongy beaks and bones

Diagnosis

- History of vitamin D deficient diet or feed
- Clinical signs of rickets and laying of thin eggs shells of the laying ducks
- Physical examination of the affected flock for signs of any deficiency disorder
- Laboratory tests like estimation of vitamin D3 level in blood of ducks.

Line of Treatment

- The dietary requirement for vitamin D3 in ducks is 200 IU/kg depending on the ratio of calcium to phosphorus. The vitamin D needs of ducks are increased several folds by inadequate levels of calcium and (or) phosphorus or by improper ratios of these minerals in the diet.
- Dry, stabilized forms of vitamin D3 are recommended to treat deficiencies
- Increase the access of the birds to sunlight.

Vitamin E Deficiency

Vitamin E deficiency causes 3 syndromes or disorders in poultry. The syndrome tends to appear individually although there are occasional overlaps between them.

The three disorders are chiefly:

1. Exudative diathesis.
2. Muscular dystrophy.
3. Encephalomalacia (crazy chick disease).

In-spite of the syndrome's association with vitamin E deficiency, each syndrome can be prevented with dietary supplementation with synthetic antioxidants, selenium and sulfur-containing amino acids, especially in case related to the prevention of exudative diathesis and muscular dystrophy.

Vitamin E deficiencies usually are seen in young chicks or turkey poults but also occur in ducklings and other poultry. Deficiencies usually occur in birds raised in closed confinement. Outbreaks commonly occur in birds fed rations that are high in polyunsaturated fats (e.g., cod liver oil, soy bean oil), that oxidize and become rancid. Vitamin E is very unstable with oxidative destruction enhanced by minerals and polyunsaturated fats in diet.

Etiology

1. Vitamin E and the selenium-containing enzyme glutathione peroxidase prevent cell membrane destruction caused by peroxides and other powerful oxidants produced as metabolic by-products.
2. There is evidence that vitamin E, selenium, and sulfur-containing amino acids perform separate functions but still act together to prevent the accumulation of harmful peroxides in tissue. Peroxides are derived, in part, from polyunsaturated acids in feeds.
3. The following facts are of interest in considering etiology:
    a. Encephalomalacia can be prevented by adding synthetic antioxidants to the feed.
    b. Exudative diathesis can be prevented by adding selenium to the feed.
    c. Muscular dystrophy can be prevented by adding cysteine, a sulfur-containing amino acid, to the feed.

Clinical Signs

- Encephalomalacia is usually seen in commercial flock fed diets with very low content of vitamin E or if an antioxidant is either omitted or is not present in sufficient quantities, or if the diet contains a reasonably high level of an unstable and unsaturated fat and is often associated with signs of ataxia , loss of balance, falling over backwards while flapping the wings, sudden prostration on the side with outstretched legs, flexed toes and head retracted .Birds that show clinical signs often continue to eat. The deficiency usually occurs between the 15th and 30th day of life; however, it may occur as early as the 7th and as late as the 56th day.
- Exudative diathesis occurs due to the deficiency of both Vitamin E and selenium in the diet of the poultry. An increased capillary permeability leads to the development of severe edema and is normally located along the ventrum of the thorax, abdomen and under the mandible. Because of

accumulation of subcutaneous fluid ventral to the abdomen birds with extensive edema have difficulty in walking and stands with their legs far apart.

- Muscular dystrophy is characterised by inapparent signs but they are mostly associated with locomotors problem. Early treatment with vitamin E through the feed or drinking water reverses the signs of exudative diathesis and muscular dystrophy due to vitamin E deficiency. Oral administration of a single dose of vitamin E (300 IU per bird) usually causes remission.

Diagnosis

1. The diagnosis can usually be made on the basis of the typical signs and gross lesions.
2. Feed analysis may indicate rancidity or likelihood of deficiency of vitamin E and/or selenium. Liver can also be analyzed for vitamin E and selenium content.
3. Gross and microscopic examination of typical lesions are valuable in confirming suspected vitamin E deficiency, especially with encephalomalacia or muscular dystrophy.

Line of Treatment

1. Recommended vitamin E levels are 30 to 150 mg/kg in the diet. The antioxidant (0.25kg of BHT or santoquin per 1000kg of feed) must be added is in the feed, if storage is long or environmental temperatures high. In the broiler chicken and turkey diets, a recommended dose of 0.3 ppm of selenium. Zero to 3 week old chicks and 0 to 6 week-old turkeys should receive half of this selenium in an organic form which is more readily available to the bird.
2. Oral administration of a single 300 IU of vitamin E per bird will often cure exudative diathesis or muscular dystrophy.
3. Birds with encephalomalacia are normally unresponsive to treatment.

Control and Prevention

1. The bird should be fed with only high-quality feed ingredients and new batches of feed should be mixed at frequent intervals. Avoid storage of mixed feeds for periods longer than 4 weeks and if prolonged storage is necessary then add chemical antioxidants.
2. Use of stabilized fats in the feed.

3. Storage of the feeds in a cool, dry place in order to reduce the vitamin and other quality losses.
4. Provide commercially prepared feeds of superior quality in their ration.

Vitamin K Deficiency

Vitamin K deficiency leads to the impairment of blood coagulation and in very severe cases it leads to the subcutaneous and internal hemorrhages which may be fatal. In the absence or the deficiency of Vitamin K, there is marked reduction of the prothrombin content in the blood and in the young chick, plasma levels are as low as 2% of normal. The prothrombin content of newly hatched chicks is only 40% that of adult birds, hence, young chicks are readily affected by a vitamin K–deficient diet. So, a deficiency of vitamin K can result in such prolonged blood clotting that severely deficient chick may bleed to death from a slight bruise or other injury. Borderline deficiency of Vitamin K causes small hemorrhagic blemishes that appears more prominently on the surface of the intestine in the breast, in the legs, wings and in the abdominal cavity.

Chicks are mostly affected and show signs of anemic due in part to loss of blood but also to development of hypoplastic bone marrow. Although blood-clotting time is a reasonable measure of the degree of vitamin K deficiency, a more accurate measure is obtained by determining the prothrombin time. Prothrombin times in severely deficient chicks may be extended from a normal of 17–20 sec to 5–6 min or longer.

Predisposing factors for vitamin K deficiency.

- Low dietary levels of the vitamin
- Low dietary levels in the maternal diet
- Lack of synthesis in the intestine
- Presence of sulfur drugs and other feed additives in the diet which suppresses the intestinal synthesis of vitamin K.
- Affection of chicks with coccidiosis where there is severe damage to the intestinal wall and can bleed excessively leading to blood loss.

Clinical signs

- Development of haemorrhages externally at areas that received abrasions such as the feet and the wings.
- Internally, presence of petechial hemorrhages in the liver and the erosion of the lining of the gizzard.
- Chicks are mostly affected and show signs of anemia.

Line of treatment

- The inclusion of menadione at 1–4 mg/ton of feed is an effective and common practice to prevent vitamin K deficiency. In case of deficiency the dose of vitamin K should be doubled.

Water Soluble Vitamins

Thiamine Deficiency (Vitamin B_1 Deficiency, Beriberi)

Thiamine deficiency occurs when there is insufficient amount of thiamine (vitamin B_1) in the duck's diet. There are two reasons for the insufficient thiamine in the duck's diet – the first being the absence or the omission of thiamine in the diet formulation and secondly due to the presence of thiaminase in the feed, which decreases the absorption of vitamin B_1 (thiamine). Some of the examples of foods containing thiaminases include milled rice, fresh fish, clams, mussels, and shrimp. Bracken fern also contains thiaminase.

The biologically active form of thiamine, Thiamine pyrophosphate, acts as a coenzyme in carbohydrate metabolism through the decarboxylation of alpha ketoacids. In cases which are suspected or showing signs of thiamine deficiency, the prompt administration of parenteral thiamine is indicated to relieve the condition.

Clinical Signs

The most common symptoms exhibited in thiamine deficiency is star-gazing /polyneuritis. Retraction of the head is due to paralysis of the anterior neck muscles. In later course, the poultry loses the ability to stand or sit upright and topple to the floor, where they may lie with heads still retracted. Birds consuming a thiamine-deficient diet soon show severe anorexia. If a severe deficiency has developed, thiamine must be force-fed or injected to induce the poultry to resume eating.

Diagnosis

- Diagnosis is mostly based on the history, the clinical signs or symptoms, the examination of the affected birds and also by the laboratory tests to determine the thiamine content.

Line of Treatment

- Administration of thiamine in their feed rations @500mg parenteral, or 100-200mg/day. It can also be added to their drinking water at 100µg/l.

Control

Modification in the diet formulation to prevent further occurrence in the flock by ensuring that the ducks are getting enough thiamine in their diet. Ducks of all ages are recommended to have 2.0 mg/kg feed or 5 mg of thiamine in their daily diet.

Riboflavin Deficiency

Riboflavin deficiency affects all the tissues although the epithelium and the myelin sheaths of some of the main nerves are the major targets of deficiency. Curled-toe" paralysis in growing chickens is one of the typical symptoms observed in riboflavin deficiency and is due to the affection in the sciatic nerves

Clinical signs

- Low egg production with low hatchability.
- Slow growth of the chicks which becomes weak and emaciated, and develop diarrhea between the first and second weeks.
- Walking on their hock joints with the aid of their wings
- The leg muscles are atrophied and flabby, and the skin is dry and harsh.
- Marked enlargement of the sciatic and brachial nerve sheaths
- Signs of riboflavin deficiency in ducks are decreased egg production, increased embryonic mortality, and an increase in size and fat content of the liver.

Line of treatment

- Treatment of the flock deficient in riboflavin can be given as two sequential daily 100-mcg doses for chicks or poults, followed by an adequate amount of riboflavin in feed.
- Due to the irreparable damage of the sciatic nerve in long standing cases of curled-toe deformity, the supplementation of riboflavin is not useful as curative.

Niacin (Nicotinic Acid) Deficiency (Vitamin B_3 Deficiency, Pellagra)

Deficiency of niacin cannot occur in chickens unless there is a concomitant deficiency of the niacin precursor, tryptophan. Unlike chickens, ducks require almost twice the amount of niacin or vitamin B_3 because of their inability to synthesize niacin from tryptophan efficiency, resulting from the presence of high amounts of enzyme, picolinic acid carboxylase in the liver. Turkeys, ducks, pheasants, and goslings are much more severely affected by niacin deficiency than are chickens. Ducklings are at risk of niacin deficiency if they are fed a poor-quality diet which does not provide enough niacin, such as feed intended for chickens.

Niacin is widely distributed in feedstuffs of both plant and animal origin. The best food sources of niacin include distiller's grains, beets, fish, various distillation and fermentation soluble, sunflower seeds and certain oilseed meals. The availability of niacin in grain and grain by-products is very low. Other sources of niacin include tablets or capsules in both regular and timed-release forms.

Clinical Signs

- Bowed legs
- Enlargement of the hock joints
- Loss of appetite and retarded growth
- Typical pigeon-toed stance
- Inability to walk and
- Weakness

Diagnosis

- History and Clinical signs.
- Physical exam of Birds.
- Feed analysis.

Line of treatment

- An allowance of 55–70 mg/kg of feed appears to be satisfactory for ducks, geese, and turkeys.
- Supplemental Niacin in diet 80-100 mg of niacin per kg of feed.

Prevention

- Feeding of commercial feed intended for waterfowl
- Niacin should be supplemented to the ducklings @ 70 mg of niacin per kg of feed and breeding ducks @50 mg of niacin per kg of feed.
- Provision of brewer's yeast as it is a good source of niacin.

Pantothenic Acid Deficiency

Pantothenic acid, also called vitamin B_5, is one of eight water-soluble B vitamins. Pantothenic acid is found in two enzymes, coenzyme A (CoA) and acyl carrier protein (ACP), and it is involved in the metabolism of carbohydrate, fat and protein. Vitamin B_5 is also important in the synthesis of red blood cells, as well as sex and stress-related hormones produced in the adrenal glands. Deficiency of this vitamin is rare in the poultry as the poultry birds receive this in their diet in the form of plant and animal origin.

Clinical signs

- Reduced egg production and marked drop in hatchability.
- Subcutaneous hemorrhages and severe edema in the embryos from hens with pantothenic acid deficiency with marked mortality in the later stage of incubation.
- Reduced growth and feed consumption, poor feathering with feathers becoming ruffled and brittle, and a rapidly developing dermatitis.
- Cornified feet and wart-like lumps occur on the balls of the feet which later leads to bacterial infection.
- Ducks do not show the usual signs noted for chickens and turkeys, except for retarded growth, but mortality can be quite high.

Most poultry diets contain supplements of calcium pantothenate. Periodically, growing chickens fed practical diets develop a scaly condition of the skin and the exact cause of which is not known.

Line of treatment

- Treatment with both calcium pantothenate (2 g) and riboflavin (0.5 g) in the drinking water (50 gal [190 L]) for a few days has been successful in some instances.
- Diets usually contain supplemental pantothenic acid at 12 mg/kg.

Vitamin B_6 Deficiency (Pyridoxine Deficiency)

Vitamin B_6, also called pyridoxine, is one of eight water-soluble B vitamins. Vitamin B_6 refers to a group of three compounds: pyridoxol (pyridoxine), pyridoxal and pyridoxamine. Vitamin B_6 is needed for normal function and development of the brain and helps the body to make the hormones serotonin and nor-epinephrine, which influence mood, and melatonin, which helps to regulate the body clock. Anemia is often noted in ducks but is seldom seen in chickens and turkeys. Anemia is likely due to a disturbance in the synthesis of proto-porphyrins. Pyridoxine is also required by several enzymes, including those involved in the breakdown of amino acids.

Clinical signs

The most common clinical signs exhibited by ducks in pyridoxine deficiency are

- Inappetence with poor growth rate.
- Chondrodystrophy.
- Exhibition of characteristic nervous behavior like jerky, nervous movements of the legs, running aimlessly about, flapping their wings, or squatting with their wings slightly spread out and their heads resting on the ground and convulsion.
- Perosis develops in border line deficiency with one leg usually being crippled and one or both middle toes bent inward at the first joint.
- In adult birds, deficiency often results in reduced appetite, leading to the reduced egg production and a decline in hatchability.

Diagnosis

- Based on the history and clinical signs.
- Feed analysis ie the diet formulation.

Line of Treatment

- Provide oral supplements of vitamin B6 or vitamin B6-rich food sources.
- Ducks and geese should receive 5-7 mg/kg of their diet in Vitamin B6.

Biotin Deficiency

Vitamin H or B7 is commonly known as Biotin, is an essential water-soluble vitamin which can be synthesized by the bacteria in the intestine. It is also available in small amounts in a number of foods.

For the regulation of the normal function of the thyroid and adrenal glands, the reproductive tract and the nervous system biotin is essential for the body. Biotin deficiency often causes abnormal cornification and keratinization of the epidermis and, thereby leading to low tensile strength and skin lacerations.

Clinical signs

- Presence of dry scaly, flaky skin along the legs and top portions of the feet.
- Callus formation at the bottom of the foot which develop deep fissures and start to bleed.
- Development of lesions around the corners of the bird's mouth which slowly spreads to the area around the beak.
- Sticky eyelids
- Young, growing chicks may develop leg deformities, consisting of perosis, crooked legs, and enlargement and twisting of the hock joint.

- Impaired muscular coordination in the young and growing chicks.
- Beak deformities, such as scissors beak and parrot beak.
- Delay in the healing of the wound.
- Increased risk of developing secondary bacterial infections anywhere where their skin is exposed, such as their feet (bumble foot) and bare patches without feathers (breast blister).
- Occurrence of fatty liver and kidney syndrome (FLKS).

Diagnosis

- Clinical signs of dry scaly legs, callus formation in legs etc
- Plasma biotin levels <100 ng/100 mL have been reported as a sign of deficiency.

Line of treatment

- Addition of 150 mg biotin/tonne of feed is essential especially when significant amounts of wheat or wheat byproducts are used in the diet.

Folic Acid (Vitamin B_9) Deficiency

Poultry birds are more susceptible to folacin deficiency than other farm animals. Folic acid deficiency mostly affects the epithelial linings, the GI tract, the epidermis, and the bone marrow, as well as cell growth and tissue regeneration. Folic acid deficiency often leads to the development of macrocytic (megaloblastic) anemia and leukopenia.

Clinical signs

- Poor feathering, slow growth, an anemic appearance and sometimes perosis. Due to anaemia there is a sign of development of a waxy-white color and pale mucous membranes in the mouth.
- Folic acid deficiency often leads to the failure of hen bird's reproductive tract development due to the severely impaired cell division.
- Macrocytic anaemia due to failure of red blood cell maturation and immune system cellular dysfunction.

Diagnosis

- The clinical signs of megaloblastic anaemia, poor feathering etc are useful in diagnosis.
- Increased erythrocyte phosphoribosyl pyrophosphate concentration can be used as a diagnostic tool in folacin-deficient chicks.

Line of treatment

- Administration of 5 mg folic acid /kg feed will return the hemoglobin values and the growth rate to normal within one week of administration in the diet.

Vitamin B_{12} Deficiency

Vitamin B_{12} is an essential part of several enzyme systems but most importantly in the metabolism of nucleic acids and proteins with most reactions involving the transfer or synthesis of methyl groups. It also functions in the carbohydrate and the fat metabolism.

Clinical signs

- Reduced weight gain and low feed intake in growing young ones, along with poor feathering and nervous disorders.
- Perosis due to the secondary effect of dietary deficiency of methionine or choline.
- Anemia, erosion of the gizzard, and fatty infiltration of the heart, liver, and kidneys.
- Reduced egg size.
- Marked reduction in the hatchability
- Changes noted in embryos from B12-deficient breeders include a general hemorrhagic condition, fatty liver, fewer myelinated fibers in the spinal cord, and high incidence of mid-term embryo deaths.

Line of treatment

Vitamin B_{12} deficiency is highly unlikely, especially for birds grown on litter or where animal-based ingredients are used and in cases of deficiency it can be treated with the provision of vitamin in their diet @ 20 mcg/g feed for 1–2 wk.

Choline Deficiency

Choline is a vitamin-like essential nutrient that serves several important functions in the duck's body. It is a essential for building and maintaining cell structure. Choline plays an essential role in multiple functions, it aids in fat metabolism in the liver, helps in the formation of acetylcholine, a substance that makes possible the transmission of nerve impulses and it also an important source of labile methyl groups.

Clinical Signs

- Reduced growth rate in young, growing duckling.
- Perosis, first characterized by pinpoint hemorrhages about the hock joint, followed by an apparent flattening of the tibio-metatarsal joint. This is followed by the Achilles' tendon slips from its condyles which is rendering the bird relatively immobile.

Diets that contain appreciable quantities of soybean meal and wheat bran are unlikely to be deficient in choline. Other sources of choline are fish meal, liver meal, meat meals, distiller's soluble and yeast. A number of commercial choline supplements are available and supplemental choline is routinely used in most poultry feeds.

Nutritional Requirements of Choline in Ducks

The choline requirement for growing ducks ranges from 750 to 2,000 mg/kg (341 to 909 mg/lb) of diet. When ducklings are methionine deficient, it markedly increases the choline requirements needed for ducks.

Diagnosis

- History & Clinical signs like the presence of perosis.
- Physical examination.
- Feed analysis or diet assessment.

Line of Treatment

- Provide choline in the diet @ 1,300-1,900 mg/kg in daily diet as supplements or choline-rich food sources.
- Supplementation of a balanced diet
- Supplement with B-vitamins after hatching.

Miscellaneous Disorders

Broken Leg (Fractured Leg)

Broken legs in a duck are considered as an emergency condition and should be treated immediately. The affected ducks usually show lameness, reluctance to walk or in some there is total absence of walking. There are also signs of swelling and discoloration at the site of injury.

Types of Bone Fractures

Four types of fractures are most commonly seen in ducks. They are:

1. Comminuted fractures: In this type there is total shattering of the bones.
2. Displaced fractures: In this type, there is misalignment of the broken bones.
3. Open or compound fractures: In this type of fracture, the bone has broken through the skin, or the initial injury has exposed the broken bone.
4. Un-displaced or hairline fractures: In this type of fracture, there is only mild fracture of the bone with no damage to the tissue surrounding it.

Clinical Symptoms

- Lameness
- Difficulty in walking and pain on palpation
- Swelling and discoloration at the site of injury.
- Reluctance to stand or walk.

Line of Treatment

Treatment will largely depend on the type and severity of the fracture. If there is very severe fracture then there will be surgical intervention to correct it.

Diagnosis

- History and clinical signs,
- Physical examination of the site of fracture
- Radiography of the affected site.

Line of Treatment

- Provide rest and isolation of the affected ducks with proper feeding and management.
- Correction of the fractured site and proper management and care of the site post surgery for proper healing to take place.

Cataracts (Cloudiness of eye)

Clouding of the eye's natural lens is known as Cataract. The oxidative changes in the duck's lens are found to be the cause for the formation of the cataract in ducks. Studies have also shown that the high intake of antioxidants and omega-3 fatty acids may help in the prevention of the development of certain types of cataracts.

In cataract, due to the inability of the light to pass through the lens there is impairment of vision which often results in blindness in the long run.

Symptoms

The symptoms that are generally manifested in this condition is cloudiness of the eye (s), the visible whiteness in the pupil and blindness.

Diagnosis

Diagnosis is mostly based on the history, the clinical signs and the observation of the symptoms on physical eye examination.

Line of Treatment

The affected flocks should be kept isolated and confined in a limited area free from the flock and proper care and management need to be done. Ensure that the birds are receiving enough riboflavin and vitamins A and E in their diet.

Cloacitis (Vent Gleet, Infected Cloaca, Pasting)

Localized inflammatory condition of the duck's vent and cloaca is known as Cloacitis or commonly called as Vent gleet. This condition mostly affects the female ducks having less access to water to bathe and is usually associated with the soiling of the vent with faeces and urates. There is presence of swelling at the site which leads to ulceration and is often associated with a foul smell.

Clinical signs

- Dull appearance of the feathers
- Presence of soiling of the vent feathers
- Decrease in the production of eggs
- Reduced appetite
- Foul smelling odour
- Inflammation of the vent area on examination and difficulty in defecation with the presence of slimy droppings.

Diagnosis

- History and clinical signs.
- Typical clinical signs like foul smelling odor concurrent with inflammation of the vent area and soiling of the vent feathers

Line of treatment

- Keep the cloaca area clean and free of built-up faeces by using a warm soapy water to wash off the buildup faeces.

- Daily dressing of the affected site with an iodine-based antiseptic (Betadine) to make sure that the cloaca area is kept clean.

Control and Prevention

- Provide a clean water source for the ducks to swim.
- Reduce the exposure of the ducks to the stressful conditions
- Provision of a balanced diet.

Egg Binding Condition

The failure of an egg to pass through the oviduct within a normal period of time is known as egg binding condition and is a commonly encountered problem in egg-laying female ducks.

Clinical Signs

This condition is generally manifested by the appearance of a swollen abdomen, constipation, lethargy, fluffed feather, penguin like stance and poor egg production.

Diagnosis

- Mostly by palpation of the egg mass on physical examination.
- Radiography confirms the presence of calcified egg.

Diagnosis

- History and clinical signs,
- Physical exam and radiography
- Ultrasonography - Useful for visualizing of the non-mineralized eggs which may be present in the oviduct behind a larger, mineralized egg.
- Serum chemistry wherein there is an elevated level of total and ionized calcium and cholesterol.

Line of Treatment

- Reduce stress to the animal and keep it in a warm and isolated place
- Give supplementation of calcium, selenium, vitamin A protein in diet in their diet.
- Surgical intervention or laparotomy is done when there is involvement of the presence of soft shells, egg fragments or adherence of the eggs to the uterus and oviduct are involved.

- Reduced light exposure as it can helps to minimize the reproductive activity.
- Warm and humid environment is helpful, so warm bath may be given to duck.
- Manual removal by applying pressure towards cloca or aspiration of egg is also helpful.

Control and Prevention

- Implantation of hormones to prevent the ducks from laying eggs.
- Provision of a balanced diet for laying ducks but care should be taken not to overdo it.

Cyst of Feather Follicle

Feather follicle cysts are a type of cyst where feather follicles are packed with fluid, semisolid or gaseous material and can develop in any tissue, but are most frequently found as hard nodules or lumps on or directly below the skin of the duck.

Common causes of cysts in ducks

- Damage to feathers.
- Genetic predisposition.
- Tumors and infections.
- Blockages of ducts in the body which cause a fluid build-up.
- Parasites and inflammation.

Asymmetric feather growth develops when the damage occurs on just one side of the follicle, in which it is not able to break through the skin resulting in the curling back within the follicle and fill with keratin, instead of producing a feather.

Clinical Signs

Presence of abnormal lumps on or directly below the skin.

Diagnosis

- History and clinical signs.
- Physical examination.
- Ultrasound and CAT scan.
- Biopsy - To confirm and rule out whether it is cancerous.

Line of Treatment

Draining or surgical removed of the cyst by the insertion of a needle or catheter into the cavity.

Traumatic Ventriculitis

Foreign objects can harm their bodies if ingested as the curious behavior of ducks often leads them to the ingestion of these foreign objects which ultimately causes impaction, inflammation, metal poisoning, peritonitis, and penetration of their gastrointestinal tract in few cases.

Ducks are particularly drawn to any shiny objects. Examples of some few are - jewelry, stones, bedding, small metal objects such as nails, nuts, washers, clips, bits of wire, screws, staples, etc., pieces of glass, wood, plastic, string, feathers, floats and lures woman's stockings trash, carpet fibers and loose change.

Clinical signs

The most common symptoms manifested on ingestion of such objects are - respiratory distress, head shaking, difficulty in swallowing feeds, inappetence, enlargement of the abdomen, weight loss and depression.

Diagnosis

- History and clinical signs.
- Physical examination.
- Video-endoscopy.
- Radiography and blood tests.

Line of Treatment

- Endoscopic removal
- Surgical intervention may be required to remove the foreign body which will cause internal damage or are toxic.

Control and Prevention

- Do not leave small metal or plastic objects where ducks have potential access.
- Carefully search and remove the presence of any small metal objects following any construction or repair of the duck's pen.
- Prevent the access of the ducks to waste area

Frostbite

It is a localized tissue injury caused by the cooling and thawing of tissues usually the featherless areas such as their legs and feet. Frostbite is most commonly seen in ducks living in colder regions; however, ducks in warmer regions left unprotected during the colder seasons are also at risk of developing frostbite.

Among the duck breeds, Muscovy ducks are found to be susceptible to frostbite along their faces. During the early stages of frostbite, initially the affected area is cold to the touch and/or may show mild redness and as the severity increases, so does the degree of inflammation with severe redness, swelling and pain in the affected sites, often spreading from the toes into the webs of feet. The advanced stages of frostbite usually appear as a shriveled and blackened tissue. There is no reversion once the tissue gets damaged and it will eventually lead to the loss of the affected tissue.

Clinical Signs

- Decreased use of affected limb and there is oedema of the affected site.
- Blackened discoloration of frostbite tissue.
- Frostbite tissue appears mummified with loss of mobility.

Diagnosis

- History and Clinical signs.
- Physical exam.

Line of Treatment

- Rapid provision of warmth to the frozen tissue in a warm (body temperature) water bath.
- Pentoxifylline: Given orally at a dosage of 15 mg/kg q8-12h for 2-6 weeks may be helpful.
- Topical application of aloe vera has been shown to significantly improve tissue survival, both alone and in combination with oral pentoxifylline.

Precautions

- Direct application of heat should be avoided.
- Rubbing of the affected areas should be avoided.
- Do not rewarm the tissue and then put the duck back outside in the cold.
- Thawing and refreezing of skin tissue will cause even more damage so should be avoided.

Gout (Avian Gout, Urate deposition)

Gout is an inflammatory disease which is caused by the accumulation of urate crystals in the joints or throughout one or more organs in the duck's body. The deposition of the urate occurs as a result of multiple factors like the impaired kidney function, impaired mechanism for the excretion of uric acid, and/or by overloading the kidneys with too much uric acid beyond the limit for the kidneys to handle.

There are two forms of gout-

1. Articular gout
2. Visceral gout

In some ducks, both visceral gout and articular gout may occur at the same time.

Articular gout

Accumulation of sodium urate crystals in the joints and synovial sheaths is known as articular gout. Articular gout is chronic in nature and sporadic in prevalence. Articular gout most commonly affects the male ducks.

Postmortem gross lesions are noted in the kidneys but in most of the cases the joints especially the feet are involved. The possible causes for the development of articular gout is because of the high protein diet, excess dietary calcium which causes kidney damage, low-phosphorus diet which leads to the formation of kidney stones, high energy diet, genetical defects and also because of the mycotoxins too.

Visceral gout

It occurs as a result of the excessive accumulation of sodium urate crystals within one or more organs, such as the kidneys, liver, heart, pericardium, and air sacs.

Visceral gout is more commonly prevalent comparing to the articular gout and is more acute in nature. it occurs both in male and female and has no gender predisposition. It can affect the whole flock at a time too unlike the articular gout which is sporadic in nature.

The postmortem gross lesions in visceral gout are mostly observed in the kidneys where there is white chalky deposit with an abnormally small sized kidney. The involvement of the joint may or may not be present. Most possible causes for the development of visceral gout is because of the following.

Severe dehydration, administering sodium bicarbonate in their diet which disturbs their urine pH, presence of an infectious agents, deficiency of vitamin

A, secondary to urolithiasis, neoplasia, immune mediated glomerulonephritis and exposure to certain toxic substances.

Clinical Signs

- Presence of swollen-warm-painful leg joints.
- Firm masses visible through the skin,
- Lameness
- Purplish darkening of the skin,
- Difficulty in walking and their reluctance to move with the presence of lethargy.

Diagnosis

- History and Clinical signs.
- Radiography
- Presence of high levels of uric acid in the blood.
- Post mortem findings.

Line of Treatment

Balanced diet with quality protein source and supplementation of vitamin A in the diet.

Control and Prevention

- Provide ducks with fresh, clean water source
- Provide ducks with vitamin A supplementation.
- Optimum level of protein in their diet.
- Customary access to the pasture grasses.

Heat Stress

The absence of sweat glands and the naturally high body temperatures (41°C/106°F) of the poultry makes them susceptible to overheating during the hot weather conditions. They naturally regulate their body in such condition only by panting which requires more energy than sweating. The heat stress leads to increased production of free radicals causes oxidative damage to lipids, proteins, and DNA in duck. Heat stress also decreases the productivity of ducks, due to the reduced intake of feeds, protein synthesis, endocrine dysfunction, less antioxidant capacity, and derangement of calcium and phosphorous balance.

Ultimately, without relief from the heat, birds will tire from heat exhaustion. The increase in respiratory rate also has an effect on the amount of ionized calcium in their body. In female laying ducks which require high amount of calcium for eggshell formation, heat stress often results development of thin-shelled or smaller eggs and/or decreased egg production.

Clinical Signs

- Excessive panting signs
- Continuously flapping of the wings up and down.
- Motionless standing for long periods of time and exhibition of abnormal restless behavior.

Diagnosis

- History and clinical signs of panting with restlessness
- Physical examination of the affected ducks

Management

- Relocate or move the ducks to a cooler place or location.
- Dip their webbed feet into a cool bath slowly.
- Placing of small ice packs under their wings for up to 60 seconds then removed it for a few minutes and repeats it again for some time.
- Provide fans, misting sprinklers, ensure receiving adequate ventilation.
- Avoid overcrowding.

Control

- Providing fresh, cool and clean water to all flock members.
- Provision of enough shade area, throughout all times of the day, for each member of the flock to go in order to get out of the sun.
- Provision of good ventilation: Birds that are in poorly ventilated areas are at a heightened risk of heat stress as it blocks air flow.
- Provision of fans and/or position the birds outside enclosure in such a way as to maximize wind exposure and good airflow.
- Proper design of the duck enclosure to minimize heat stress.

Keel Bone Injuries

Keel bone injuries in ducks results in pain and discomfort in the area of the keel. Bruising, abscess, dislocation, or fracture (brake) of the keel may result due to the injuries.

Etiology

There are several causes that lead to the injury of the keel in ducks. The most common ones being -

- Hitting the keel on hard or rough surface repeatedly.
- Repetitive friction against the keel.
- Direct impact or trauma to the keel.
- Prolonged resting on the keel, especially in unsanitary conditions.

Clinical Signs

- Thinning of the feather.
- Reddening of the skin.
- Presence of wound.
- Tenderness and bruising of the keel.

Diagnosis

- History and Clinical signs.
- Physical examination.

Line of Treatment

- Administering of oral antibiotics and anti-inflammatory to control the infection.
- Thorough cleaning and disinfection of the wound
- Topical application of antibiotics, such as silver sulfadiazine cream.
- In severe cases, debridement surgery may be needed.

Prevention

- Use of a soft, padded surfaces such as rubber mats.
- Application or use of a 'donut' therapy device or rolled up cloth formed into a ring, to protect the duck's keel.
- Exercise trauma prevention.

Leech Infestation

Leech infestation has been reported to occur in ducks. It should be considered an emergency condition and can be rapidly fatal to the bird. Leeches are visible to the naked eye however they may go undetected if they have already migrated inside of the duck. Usually, they are seen protruding out of the duck's eyes (the conjunctiva just below the nictitating membrane) or from the nares. Infested ducks will usually appear distressed and irritated. They may frequently shake their heads and try cleaning their bill in the water, in an attempt to remove the leeches from their face. If leeches are feeding in the area around the eyes, affected ducks will usually also show signs of conjunctivitis and keratitis, possibly resulting in blindness. When the nasal cavity is affected, bleeding may occur from the duck's nostrils. Secondary infections caused by leeches are common.

Symptoms

- Vigorous head shaking.
- Signs of distress and discomfort.
- Conjunctivitis and Blindness.

Diagnosis

- History and Clinical signs.
- Physical examination.

Treatment and management

- Manual removal of the leeches using forceps, after applying proxymetacaine hydrochloride to the surface to aid in removal.
- Ivermectin: Dipping the ends of the protruding leeches in ivermectin (10 ug/ml), apply in the form of nasal drops, or administer 0.02 ml/kg orally or subcutaneous.
- Ophthalmic antibiotic ointment to prevent secondary bacterial infections involving the eyes.

Photosensitization

The ingestion or a direct contact with certain photosensitive-causing plants or medications induces photosensitization. Photosensitization is an inflammatory skin condition induced by ultraviolet (UV) light exposure. Ducks are very sensitive to photosensitization especially on their non-feathered areas of the body, such as on their webbed feet, legs, eyes and bill.

The following plants have been reported to cause photosensitization in ducks -

- Parsley (*Petroselinum sativum*)
- Bishop's weed (*Ammi majus*)

- Toothpickweed (*Ammi visnaga*)
- *Cymopterus longipes:* The two phototoxic furocoumarins, oxypeucedanin and isoimperitorin, causes severe acute photosensitization in ducks upon exposure to sunlight.
- *Cymopterus watsonii:* The leaves and seeds of the spring parsley plant contains furocoumarinas, which cause acute photosensitization in ducks. The affected birds in later stage may develop deformalities of legs, beak, comb and wattle as well as reduced eyesight.
- Hypericum spp. Berries
- Giant hogweed (*Heracleum mantegazzianum*): Giant hogweed causes photosensitivity upon contact and subsequent exposure to sunlight. The leaves and roots have the highest concentrations of toxins during the early part of the growing season. It causes blindness when it affects their eyes and also leads to severe crippling deformities to their beak and feet.

Clinical Signs

- Chronic lesions of the beak, foot web and eyes.
- Sticky eyelids, redness of eyes and blindness.

Diagnosis

- History and clinical signs.
- Physical examination.
- Radiographs and laboratory tests.

Management

- Isolate the bird from the flock and place in a safe, comfortable, warm with easy access to water and food.
- Reduce the exposure of the ducks to sunlight for at least 3 days following ingestion or contact with photosensitive plants.

Prevention

- Don't allow ducks access to plants which are known to cause photo-sensitivity in ducks.
- Do not feed parsley to ducks.

Perosis (Slipped Tendon)

Slipped tendon, also known as perosis, occurs when the duck's Achilles (gastrocnemius) tendon pops off the side of the bone, resulting in pain and reluctance to put weight on the leg.

The condition can be reversed if detected in the early developing stage. It is easily confused with splay leg and rickets however with splay leg, the whole leg deviates rather than just at the hock and in rickets, it is caused by the long bone deformity and not due to the tendon displacement.

Clinical Signs

- There is a sudden onset of lameness with the manifestation of leg rotation.
- There is presence of swelling over the back point of the hock.
- Difficulty in walking.
- The affected bird shows an increased amount of time laying down.
- Intermittent severe lameness with interposed periods of mild lameness.
- An intermittent popping sound may be heard each time the tendon dislocates.

Diagnosis

- History and clinical signs.
- Physical examination and radiography.

Management

- Isolate the affected bird from the flock and provide warm bedding with easy access to water and food.
- Supplement manganese in their diet while ensuring not to provide excess calcium.
- Fix the splinting to provide the duckling support and stabilization.
- Antibiotics and anti-inflammatory medications to be administered to the affected duck.

Control

- Don't feed excessive calcium, as it can cause manganese deficiency.
- Ensure adult ducks that are intended to be used for breeding purposes are receiving enough manganese in their diet and not excessive calcium.

Splay Leg (Spraddle leg)

Splay leg, also known as spraddle leg, is a type of leg deformity that is usually seen in young, newly hatched ducklings.

It is most commonly caused by raising ducklings on a ground surface that does not provide adequate traction, however it can also be the result of problems during incubation, and less commonly genetics. Splay legs may affect one or both the legs and it may differ in its severity from mild to severe. The condition is characterized by the legs splaying outward or laterally from underneath the duckling's body.

Corrective orthopedic techniques and physical therapy are used for the correction of the splay. The main purpose of all this treatment procedure is to ensuring the legs are in the correct distance apart and are not too tight as to restrict blood circulation to the leg, nor too loose so that it is ineffective.

Clinical Signs

- Inability to stand properly.
- One or both legs splaying outward.
- Difficult in walking.

Diagnosis

- History and clinical signs.
- Physical examination.

Line of Treatment

- Hydrotherapy.
- An alternative orthopedic device that uses a foam block with holes cut at the appropriate distance apart for the legs.

Control and Prevention

- Ensure that ducklings are raised on non-slippery surface.
- Do not place incubators in rooms where they receive direct sunlight.

Sticky Eye

An eye infection in ducks can be caused by a number of causes like the presence of debris, a scratch or rough mating. In ducks, eye issues and respiratory issues go hand in hand as their sinuses run down the back of their head.

Clinical Signs

- Closed eye, bubbling eye, redness or tearing.

Line of Treatment

- Cleansing of the ducks eye with saline water and then giving access to a nice, deep water bowl to submerge her entire head can often clear up the problem.

- In more serious infection a natural camphor-based solution can be added to the water or applied to the nostrils to relieve the symptoms.

Impacted Crop

Ducks sometimes suffer from an impacted crop as they have the habit of practically eating everything, they get hold of and suffer mostly from impaction when they consume long pieces of string, twine, plastic or even rubber band.

Common causes of impaction of crop-

- Straw and long blades of grass
- String like hay bale twine, artificial grass, carpet fiber, etc.
- Feathers
- Bedding (mulch, wood chips)
- Skins from fruits like bananas or persimmons
- Small plastic or metal objects
- Raw oats or rice, which swell with water

Clinical signs: Anorexia

Line of Treatment

- Normally, the crop of a duck is usually empty in the morning since ducks digest everything they eat overnight, so in case of a suspicion of an impacted crop, gentle massaging of the crop.
- Providing grit, some olive oil and plenty of water to the duck will help in relieving the impaction.

Control

- To prevent the occurrence of this proper cutting of the chaff needs to be done.

Prolapsed Penis/Vent

A prolapsed vent or a penis in ducks occurs when a portion of the oviduct prolapsed outside of the duck's body while she's laying an egg, or the drake's penis doesn't retract back after mating. In both the conditions normally, it gets corrected on its own but it's important to keep the area clean, and keep it soft.

The best way to manage such cases is to isolate the affected flock and prevent it from mating and give proper diet or nutrition and plenty of room for exercise.

Wet Feather

Wet feather is a condition that occurs when a duck's feathers become water-logged and lose their ability to repel water. Loss of waterproofing on their feathers also affects a duck's ability to float. This is because their feathers are made up of tiny barbs which latch together similar to Velcro. This creates a balloon-like effect which traps air between the feathers and the skin, resulting in the formation of air bubbles. The air bubbles are what add to a duck's natural buoyancy. A duck with wet feather has an increased risk of drowning because of the affect it has on their ability to float in the water and can also cause them to get chilled and get sick.

Wet feathers are most commonly seen in ducks which are kept in an unsanitary, excessively muddy environment without access to fresh water to bathe in. Preen gland infection, lice infestation, sooty black mold, and/or contamination of their feathers with oil-based products or detergent are also some of the predisposing factors for the ducks to develop wet feathers.

The best way to prevent the occurrence of this is to provide regular access to clean, fresh water to bathe or swim in, maintaining a clean and dry living environment and avoiding the application of any oil-based products to their feathers.

Feather Pecking and Cannibalism in Ducks

Major problems in ducks, and again the causes are unclear. There are some differences among duck breeds in the type of injurious pecking behavior that is most frequently observed.

Anecdotal reports suggest that feather picking and feather pecking follow a seasonal pattern, occurring more frequently in spring and fall. Unlike in Pekin ducks, cannibalism is a major issue for Muscovy ducks. This cannibalism in Muscovy ducks is not supported by the redirected foraging hypothesis, as it is in chickens. Thus far, research has found that outbreaks of cannibalism in Muscovy ducks can occur as early as 13 days of age and seem to be related to the appearance of new feathers.

Cannibalism is defined as the pecking, tearing, and consuming of skin, tissue, or organs of flock mates. It is a problem that can occur among birds of any age and of any breed. Cannibalism can affect many different types of poultry, including chickens, ducks, turkeys, quail, and pheasants. Cannibalism can occur in all types of housing systems, including cages, floor pens, aviaries, and free-range systems.

Cannibalism is a learned behaviour that can spread quickly through a flock. Poultry have a tendency to imitate each other, so when one member of the flock begins aggressive pecking, others will follow suit. If cannibalism is not closely monitored, the resulting losses to the flock due to flesh injuries and death can be quite high. Cannibalism is easier to prevent than to treat. The cause has a genetic component, but management conditions play a major role as well. Outbreaks can occur in even the well-managed flock, but problems are less likely to occur if preventive measures are in place.

Causes

- Overcrowding precipitates feather pecking and cannibalism in ducks.
- A high temperature in the poultry house causes the birds to become uncomfortable and prone to pecking.
- Extremely bright lights or excessively long periods of light will cause the birds to become hostile toward each other and influences cannibalistic behaviour.
- Cannibalism outbreaks can be initiated by the injury of one bird and subsequent pecking of the injury by a flock or cage mate as they are attracted to blood.
- The act of cannibalism increases with the intermixing of birds of different ages, breeds, colours, or sizes that have not been reared together as it disturbs the social order and promotes pecking.
- Unexpected changes in managemental practices and environmental stress lead to aggression and development of cannibalism.
- The everted cloaca is highly attractive for pecking as a result of which cannibalism outbreaks begins.

Control and Prevention

- Selecting genetic stock that is not prone to cannibalism.
- Separate birds doing the severe feather pecking directed at injuries or vents of other birds.
- Take out victims of cannibalism and care separately or cull.
- Dim lights to an intensity of 0.5 to 1.0 foot-candles.
- Adequate feed and water space along with perched housing environment.
- For laying ducks add more nest boxes.
- Regular beak trimming.

Ascites Syndrome in Duck (Water Belly)

It is a condition where there is an accumulation of non inflammatory transudate in one or more of the peritoneal cavities or potential spaces. Ascites may result from increased vascular hydraulic pressure, vascular damage, increased tissue oncotic pressure, or decreased vascular oncotic (usually colloidal) pressure, but is most commonly associated with venous hypertension resulting from right heart failure in response to increased pulmonary resistance. Ascites, or water belly, is a common condition in ducks. The accumulation of fluids in the abdominal cavity is usually associated with the interference of the blood circulation through the liver.

The most common cause of ascites is increased vascular hydraulic pressure in the venous system, which most commonly is caused by right ventricular failure (RVF), also associated with hepatic fibrosis. Pulmonary hypertension occurs frequently in chicken secondary to high altitude-associated hypoxia with resultant polycythemia and increased blood viscosity. It also occurs frequently secondary to the RBC rigidity of sodium toxicity and less frequently from lung pathology. When ascites occurs at high altitudes in meat-type chickens, which have a high metabolic oxygen requirement, it is usually caused by primary or spontaneous pulmonary hypertension because of insufficient capacity of the pulmonary capillaries. Cold stress, even briefly, during the first 3 wk of life is known to markedly increase predisposition to ascites syndrome.

Amyloidosis of the liver is also responsible for the development of ascites in both meat-type ducks and breeders.

Pathogenesis

Pulmonary hypertension syndrome develops when there is an exertion of the heart to pump more blood through the lungs to meet the body's oxygen requirement thereby increasing the pressure in the pulmonary arteries. The resultant volume and pressure overload on the right ventricle causes the dilatation and hypertrophy of the right ventricular wall, valvular insufficiency, RVF and ultimately leads to ascites. Bird lungs are rigid and fixed in the thoracic cavity. Lung size in proportion to body weight, and particularly to muscle mass, decreases as meat-type ducks grow. Increased blood flow results in primary pulmonary hypertension and cor pulmonale with sporadic cases of RVF and ascites in birds as in the birds, the expansion of the capillaries is minimal so they are unable to accommodate the increased blood flow.

Clinical signs

Affected duck have abdominal distensions caused by the accumulation of the ascetic fluid and are reluctant to move and are cyanotic and dyspneic. Because growth stops as RVF develops, affected birds are comparatively smaller than their pen mates. However, rapid growth rate is a known predisposing factor, and sometimes the largest birds are affected, with occurrence in males more frequent than in females. The ascites increases the respiratory rate and reduces exercise tolerance. Frequently die on their backs. Not all the birds affected by pulmonary hypertension syndrome will develop ascites as some birds may die suddenly even before the development of the ascites.

Diagnosis

Post mortem lesion of an enlarged heart; enlarged, thickened right ventricle; or fluid in the body cavities and heart sac. Enlarged or thickened right ventricle is suggestive of pulmonary hypertension syndrome, even if there is no fluid in the body or heart sac.

Management & Control

- Reducing feed density or availability thereby reducing the birds' metabolic oxygen requirement.
- Environmental temperature, humidity, and air movement should be controlled to prevent excessive loss of body heat, particularly in the early neonatal period.
- Other etiologic factors (eg, sodium, lung damage, liver damage, etc) that trigger ascites can be prevented by avoiding the etiologic agents involved.

Toxins and Poisoning in Ducks

Ducks are particularly susceptible to certain toxins, and in some cases strikingly more than chickens or turkeys. Therefore, proper management of ducks by the caretakers must be especially taken care of by not allowing the consumption or exposure to these toxins. Some of the most commonly encountered toxicosis and poisoning in ducks are discussed in this chapter.

Aflatoxin Poisoning

Poisoning of the ducks from ingestion of aflatoxins in the contaminated food or feed. Aflatoxins are produced by the molds *Aspergillus flavus* and *Aspergillus parasiticus*. Duck, is the most susceptible poultry species to be affected by aflatoxin . Very small amounts will cause high mortality. There are four main aflatoxins which is of concern for its toxicity - aflatoxin B1 (AFB1), B2 (AFB2), G1 (AFG1), and G2 (AFG2); AFB1 is the most common and the most biologically active. Both acute and chronic aflatoxicosis can occur, however the chronic form is the most prevalent which occurs as a result of prolonged intake of low levels of aflatoxins in a duck's diet. The adverse effect of aflatoxins depends on the age, species, nutritional status of ducks as well as the dose and length of time it was consumed.

Clinical signs

- Decreased growth rate and poor feed conversion because of the metabolites of aflatoxins bind to DNA and RNA of the cells and hence reduce protein synthesis.
- Immunosuppressive effect due to decrease cell mediated immunity and to lesser extent humoral immunity leading to vaccination failure and decrease resistance to infectious disease.
- Passage of undigested food in the dropping.
- Stunted growth,
- Anaemia of the infected birds and decreased PCV.
- Decrease egg production and decreased hatchability due to embryonic mortality.
- The primary site of toxicity of aflatoxins is the liver. There is hepatic lesions and enlargement of the liver as well as fatty liver.

Diagnosis

- History and clinical symptoms.
- Serum biochemical analysis, CBC, and coagulation testing.
- Post-mortem examination of the dead birds.
- Chemical analysis of the feed.

Control and Prevention

- Use mycotoxin-binding adsorbents.
- Use of herbal extracts like turmeric, garlic and asafetida have shown to counteract aflatoxicosis in animals and poultry through their antioxidant activity.
- Supplementation of additional levels of riboflavin, pyridoxine, folic acid and choline and increasing the crude protein content showed protective effect against aflatoxicosis.
- Antioxidants like BHT and l-napthoflavone, vitamin C and vitamin E offer protection against aflatoxin induced genotoxicity in in-vitro studies.

Toxicity of Blue-Green Algae (Phycotoxicosis)

It is seen in ducks when they ingest the water that is contaminated with cyanotoxins, during harmful algal blooms (HABs). Blooms occur most commonly in nutrient-rich, warm, bodies of water with little movement or mixing in layers. Direct intoxication with cyanotoxins occur after direct exposure to the harmful cyanobacteria, or cyanotoxin-contaminated food or water whereas the indirect effects of blooms cause an increased risk of botulism, resulting from a decrease in dissolved oxygen and the proliferation of *Clostridium botulinum*.

Present global climate change and increased CO_2 concentrations which have resulted in an increased frequency of blooms occurring worldwide and thereby an increased toxication of the ducks.

Cyanotoxins are essentially endotoxins and are generally classified into hepatotoxins, neurotoxins, dermatotoxins and cytotoxin. In most cases of poisoning, ducks are usually found dead, due to the potency of the toxin.

Symptoms

- Hypersalivation and regurgitation of the algae.
- Diarrhea and excessive thirst.
- Neurological signs viz. tremors, ataxia, wing and leg peresis with intermittent seizures.
- Reduced responsiveness and marked lethargy.
- Dilation of cutaneous vessels.
- Recumbency
- Cyanosis, open mouth breathing and sudden death.

Diagnosis

- History and clinical signs.
- Physical examination.
- Necropsy findings.
- Cyanobacteria testing of water samples.

Treatment

Administration of activated charcoal orally. Rehydration therapy along with vitamin supplementation. Antitoxins are to be used.

Lead Poisoning (Plumbism)

All species of birds are susceptible to lead poisoning and it is considered as one of the most commonly reported toxic conditions in both wild and domestic ducks especially in the waterfowls. Chickens are more resistant than the waterfowls.

There are multiple possible sources for lead toxicity as lead is widespread in the environment. In the wild ducks, it is often caused by the lead shotgun pellets or the contaminated sediments. Backyard and free-range ducks mostly pick up lead from the paint chips, lead batteries or other lead objects.

Lead poisoning can occur as an acute or chronic condition. Most lead poisoning in birds is chronic in nature which often occurs slowly, over time. Upon the ingestion of the toxin by the duck, it gets retained in the gizzard where it is grounded down and then absorbed slowly into the bloodstream where it leads to the pansystemic damage, particularly to the gastrointestinal nervous, renal and hematopoietic systems.

Clinical Signs

Clinical disease in the chronic form is usually manifested by signs of wasting, ataxia, lameness or paralysis, head tilting, circling, convulsions, blindness and anemia. In acute cases, weakness, prostration, anorexia and anemia maybe prominently observed. There is also signs of greenish diarrhea which may be due to the direct effect of the lead on the gastrointestinal and the nervous systems.

Diagnosis

Diagnosis is based on the history, clinical signs, physical exam, radiographs and laboratory tests. In hematology examination, basophilic stippling and abnormal erythrocytes are present but not observed in all the affected birds. The final diagnosis of lead poisoning is based on the level of lead content in the blood and the tissue samples. A blood lead level greater than 4 ppm wet weight, a liver lead level greater than 18ppm wet weight or a 20 ppm wet weight in kidney is considered as diagnostic.

Treatment

Treatment will depend on the level of toxicity - acute or chronic. Treatment is focused firstly on the supportive care, prevention of further exposure to the source and their further absorption in the system.

Supportive care mostly includes the control of the nervine symptoms and correcting anemia and anorexia by administration of fluids and nutritional support. Includes anticonvulsants (midazolam or diazepam given at 0.5 mg/kg IV, IM, or IN), fluid therapy, chelation, nutritional support, and antibiotics/antifungals. Regular laboratory testing and assessment during and after treatment should be done.

The following chelators can be used -

D, Swayne., J, Glisson., L, McDougald., L, Nolan., D, Suarez., V, Nair. (2013). Diseases of Poultry Wiley-Blackwell.

da Silva JF, Peluzio JM, Prado G, Madeira JE, Silva MO, de Morais PB, Rosa CA, Pimenta RS, Nicoli JR. (2015). Use of Probiotics to Control Aflatoxin Production in Peanut Grains. ScientificW d'Ovidio, Dario, Emilio Noviello, and Chiara Adami Nerve stimulator-guided sciatic-femoral nerve block in raptors undergoing surgical treatment of pododermatitis Veterinary anaesthesia and analgesia.

Dos, Anjos, F.R., Ledoux, D.R., Rottinghaus, G.E., Chimonyo, M. (2015). Efficacy of adsorbents (bentonite and diatomaceous earth) and turmeric (*Curcuma longa*) in alleviating the toxic effects of aflatoxin in chicks Br Poult Sci.

DSM in Animal Nutrition & Health DSM Vitamin Supplementation Guidelines 2011 DSM (2017)

Egyed, M. N., Shlosberg, A., Eilat, A. (1975). The susceptibility of young chickens, ducks, and turkeys to the photosensitizing effect of Ammi visnaga seeds. Avian Dis.

Fiorello, C.V. (2017). Intravenous regional antibiotic perfusion therapy as an adjunctive treatment for digital lesions in seabirds J Zoo Wildl Med.

Flinchum, Gwen, BS, MS, DVM (2014). Management of Waterfowl Clinical Avian Medicine. Vol. 2.

G, Flinchum. (2014). Management of Waterfowl Clinical Avian Medicine. Vol. 18

Gabarrou, J.F., Salichon, M, R., Guy, G., Blum, J, C. (1996). Hybrid ducks overfed with boiled corn develop an acute hepatic steatosis with decreased choline and polyunsaturated fatty acid level in phospholipids. Reprod Nutr Dev.

Gholami-Ahangaran, M., M. S. S. Firouzabadi, and M. S. Firouzabadi. (2012) Evaluation of antiseptic role of one nanosilver based drug as a new therapeutic method for treatment of bumblefoot in pheasant (Phasianus colchicus). Global Veterinaria 8.1.

González, M. S., and Carrasco, D. C. (2016) Emergencies and Critical Care of Commonly Kept Fowl Veterinary Clinics of North America: Exotic Animal Practice.

Greenacre, Cheryl, B. (2015). Musculoskeletal diseases Backyard Poultry Medicine and Surgery: A Guide for Veterinary Practitioners. Wiley-Blackwell, Ames, IA, 2015. 145-159.

Gries CL, Scott ML. (1972). The pathology of thiamin, riboflavin, pantothenic acid and niacin deficiencies in the chick., *J Nutr.*

Hegsted, D.M. (1946). Nutritional studies with the duck; niacin deficiency. J Nutr.

Hochleithner, Manfred, and Claudia Hochleithner. (1996). Surgical treatment of ulcerative lesions caused by automutilation of the sternum in psittacine birds journal of Avian Medicine and Surgery.

Hong, Cai, and Feng Zeguang. (1997). Experimental Pathology of Manganese (Mn) deficiency and effects of higher phosphorus upon manganese deficiency in broiler ducks ACTA Veterinaria et *Zootechnica sinica.*

Humphreys, P.N. Wet-feather associated with Holomenopon leucoxanthum in a duck. Vet Rec. (1975)

Hu Y, Zhang J, Kong W, Zhao G, Yang M. (2017). Mechanisms of antifungal and anti-aflatoxigenic properties of essential oil derived from turmeric (*Curcuma longa* L.) on Aspergillus flavus. Food Chem.

J, Wellehan, DVM, M,S. (2003). Frostbite in Birds: Pathophysiology and Treatment Compendium October 2003.

Keymer, I. F. (1980). Disorders of the avian female reproductive system. Avian Pathology.

Lang, D, C. (1969). Infestation of ducklings with leeches. Vet Rec.

Latymer, E, A., Coates, M, E. (1981). The influence of microorganisms and of stress on the chick's requirement for pantothenic acid.. Br J Nutr.

Ma ,X., Lin ,Y., Zhang ,H., Chen, W., Wang, S.,, Ruan, D., Jiang, Z. (2014). Heat stress impairs the nutritional metabolism and reduces the productivity of egg-laying ducks. Animal Reproductive Science.

Masse, P. G., et al. (1996). Pyridoxine deficiency affects biomechanical properties of chick tibial bone Bone

Meyerholz, David K., et al. (2005). Surveillance of amyloidosis and other diseases at necropsy in captive trumpeter swans (*Cygnus buccinator*). Journal of veterinary diagnostic investigation.

Mingliang, Ling. (2005). Comparative Experiment on Typical Drugs for Mitigating Fowl Gout Caused by High-Protein Feed China Poultry.

Motzok, I., and H. D. Branion. (1948). The vitamin D requirements of growing ducks. Poultry Science

Naguib, Mark. (2017). Avian radiography and radiology. Part 1 Companion Animal 22.8

Nasr, Mohammed, A.F, et al. (2015). The effects of two non-steroidal anti-inflammatory drugs on the mobility of laying hens with keel bone fractures. Veterinary anaesthesia and analgesia

Ness, Robert D. and Jörg Mayer. (2017). Laser Therapy for Birds Laser Therapy in Veterinary Medicine: Photobiomodulation.

Nutrient Requirements of Poultry: Ninth Revised Edition. Subcommittee on Poultry Nutrition, National Research Council (1994)

Perelman, B., & Kuttin, E. S. (1988). Parsley-induced photosensitivity in ostriches and ducks Avian Pathology

QI, Xin-yong, et al. (2008). Comparative Observation of the Pathology of Chicken and Duck Gout Progress in Veterinary Medicine.

Rigdon, R. H. (1966). Hereditary myopathy in the white Pekin duck Annals of the New York Academy of Sciences.

Rodenburg, T. B., et al. (2005). Welfare of ducks in European duck husbandry systems. *World's Poultry Science Journal*

Rollinson, H.l. et al., (1950). Deaths in young ducklings associated with infestations of the nasal cavity with leeches. *Vet Rec.*

Schmidt, R. E., Reavill, D. R., & Phalen, D. N. (2015) Pathology of pet and aviary birds John Wiley & Sons.

Shaw, S. N., D'Agostino, J. J., Davis, M. R., & McCrae, E. A. (2012). Primary feather follicle ablation in common pintails (*Anas acuta*) and a white-faced whistling duck (*Dendrocygna viduata*). *Journal of Zoo and Wildlife Medicine*

Shi, D., Liao, S., Guo, S., Li, H., Yang, M., Tang, Z. (2015). Protective effects of selenium on aflatoxin B1-induced mitochondrial permeability transition, DNA damage, and histological alterations in duckling liver. Biol Trace Elem Res.

Shlosberg, A., & Egyed, M. N. (1978). Photosensitization in ducklings induced by seeds of *Cymopterus watsonii* and *C. longipes*. Avian Diseases.

Speckmann, G., and J. W. Luther. (1974). Visceral gout and amyloidosis in a mute swan (Cygnus olor) The Canadian Veterinary Journal.

Sun, L, H., Zhang, N, Y., Sun, R, R., Gao, X., Gu, C., Krumm, C, S., Qi, D, S. (2015). A novel strain of Cellulosimicrobium funkei can biologically detoxify aflatoxin B1 in ducklings. Sun LH, Zhang NY, Sun RR, Gao X, Gu C, Krumm CS, Qi DS.

Valsala, K. V., et al. (1980). Pathology of gout in ducks Kerala Journal of Veterinary Science.

Wen, Z, G., Hou, S, S., Tang, J., Feng, Y, L., Huang,W, Guo, Y,M., Xie ,M (2014) Choline requirements of male White Pekin ducks from 21 to 42 d of age. *Br Poult Sci.*

Wen, Z, G., Tang, J., Hou, S, S., Guo, Y, M., Huang, W., Xie, M. (2014). Choline requirements of White Pekin ducks from hatch to 21 days of age. Poult Sci.

Wen, Z. G., et al (2016). Effects of Dietary Methionine Levels on Choline Requirements of Starter White Pekin Ducks Asian. Australasian Journal of Animal Sciences.

Wu LS, Wu CL, Shen TF. (1984). Niacin and tryptophan requirements of mule ducklings fed corn and soy-based diets. *Poult Sci.*

Xie M, Tang J, Wen Z, Huang W, Hou S. Effects of pyridoxine on growth performance and plasma aminotransferases and homocysteine of white pekin ducks. Asian-Australas J Anim Sci. (2014)

Yiru Dong A. (2019). Thesis on injurious pecking behavior of pekin ducks on commercial farms:characteristics, development and duck welfare. Faculty of Purdue. December.

Yokoyama, R., et al. (2000). An outbreak of cataracts in layer hens accompanied by persistent decreased egg production Journal of the Japanese Society of Poultry Diseases.

Zeng T, Li JJ, Wang DQ, Li GQ, Wang GL, Lu LZ. (2014). Effects of heat stress on antioxidant defense system, inflammatory injury, and heat shock proteins of Muscovy and Pekin ducks: evidence for differential thermal sensitivities. Cell Stress Chaperones.

Zeyuan, Zhu, Shen Aihua, and Bao Chenyu. (1999). The Effects of Dietary Niacin Levels on Growth Performance and Lipid Metabolism at Later Stage of Ducklings Animal Husbandry & Veterinary Medicine.

Zhu,W., Jiang, W., Wu, LY. (2014) Dietary L-arginine supplement alleviates hepatic heat stress and improves feed conversion ratio of Pekin ducks exposed to high environmental temperature. Journal of Animal Physiology and Animal Nutrition.

unique capacity to infect and cause disease in domestic ducks and wild birds. It producing a range of syndromes including asymptomatic respiratory and digestive tract infections; systemic disease to brain, heart and pancreas and severe disseminated infection and death.

Clinical signs

The incubation period varies from few days to more than 21 days. In general, most of the avian Influenza A viruses are low pathogenic and the occurrence of such low pathogenic avian influenza A viruses cause few signs of diseases in the associated aquatic wild bird species, like ruffled feathers and reduction in laying of eggs while high pathogenic avian influenza A may exhibit the clinical signs of laboured breathing, increased recumbency and neurological signs of torticollis, circling, loss of balance and head tremor.

Necropsy findings

The common gross lesions observed in birds affected with highly pathogenic influenza virus includes inflammation of the sinuses, trachea and air sacs, ecchymosis of shank and feet, oedematous head, discoloration of the skin, haemorrhages in ovary and oviduct, enlargement of spleen and ulcers in gastro-entestinal systems.

Diagnosis

The disease is diagnosed based on the clinical signs and detection of virus by polymerase chain reaction (PCR) or real time PCR in which nucleic acid from blood or tissue samples are analysed. The virus isolation and controlled laboratory challenge of experimental birds of the same group is also used for the diagnosis of bird flu. The serological diagnosis shall be made, based on AGID, HI tests and ELISA tests.

Differential Diagnosis

It should be differentiated from diseases of ducks having similar clinical signs and symptoms like new duck disease, duck cholera, duck plague and duck viral hepatitis.

Treatment

There is no specific treatment for avian influenza in ducks and other birds.

Prevention and Control

The affected birds with clinical symptoms should be disposed of immediately following all precautionary measures. The person dealing with infected birds must wear gloves and spectacles to avoid accidental spilling of secretions or discharges from the ducks/geese. The contacts between aquatic ducks or any aquatic wild birds and domestic poultry should be avoided as water fowls acts as natural reservoirs of this viral infection. The strict biosecurity measures must be followed in farms.

Musky Duck Parvo Virus Infection

Musky duck parvovirus is caused by parvo virus and characterized by high mortality in young duckling, profuse white diarrhoea, swollen red eyelids and ascites in later stage. Muscovy ducks and several hybrid duck breeds are also susceptible to parvovirus that has been shown to be antigenically related to goose parvovirus.

Etiology

Musky duck parvovirus is a member of the family Parvoviridae and based on phylogenetic analysis it is closely related to goose parvovirus.

Epidemiology

It is highly contagious and fatal disease of Muscovy ducklings, hybrid duck breeds and goslings which causes very high mortality. The Muscovy duck parvovirus reported among Muscovy ducks in California. The young once is highly susceptible to parvo virus infection.

Transmission

The main mode of transmission is oro-faecal route as virus is excreted in large amounts in the faeces of infected birds ensuing quick spread by contact. The susceptible duckling may get infection through eggs laid by infected breeder Muscovy ducks.

Pathogenesis

The duckling gets infection through oral route or by infected eggs. After primary infection, the virus replicates in the intestine then causes transient viraemia. After viraemia virus reaches the various organs like heart, liver, kidney etc and develop various pathological changes.

Clinical findings

The clinical signs and course of disease varied in ducklings and goslings according to their age. The birds of less the 1 week of age shows rapid course of disease and death occurs in 2-5 days with major clinical signs of anorexia. In hatchery mortality may reach upto 100%. The adult birds are characterized with clinical signs of oculo-nasal discharge, profuse white diarrhoea, weakness, red and swollen eyelids and uropygial glands. In later stage birds may show retarded growth, loos of feather, reddening of skin. The accumulation of ascitic fluid in the abdomen may cause "Penguin-like" posture. The adult birds do not show any clinical signs.

Necropsy findings

Gross examination reveals fibrinous pseudo-membrane over tongue and oral cavity, perihepatitis, pericarditis, pulmonary edema, liver dystrophy, rounded apex of heart and catarrhal enteritis. The microscopic lesions show Cowdry type-A intranuclear inclusion bodies and degenerative changes in myocardium.

Diagnosis

The diagnosis may be done based on age group affected, clinical signs, course of disease and post mortem findings in field conditions. The confirmatory diagnosis can be based on isolation of the parvovirus in cell cultures or embryonated eggs from susceptible geese and muscovy ducks. The electron microscopy, immunofluorescence, ELISA, Virus neutralization, agar gel precipitation and PCR may be useful in diagnosis of disease.

Differential diagnosis

It should be differentiated from duck viral enteritis, Duck viral hepatis, *Riemerella anatipestifer* and *Pasteurella multocida infections.*

Treatment

There is no specific treatment while antimicrobials may be helpful in prevention of secondary bacterial infections. The administration of immune serum may be effective.

Prevention

The ducks free from Musky duck parvo virus infection should only be used for breeding purpose. The eggs and duckling should only procure from the country which is free from parvo virus infection.

Duck Pox

It is a sporadic infectious disease of ducks and chicken caused by Avian pox virus and characterized by wart like pox lesions in the head, oral cavity and other featherless parts of the body. Duck pox virus is different from fowl pox and pigeon pox.

Etiology

The pox virus is a DNA virus with complex symmetry belongs to the family poxviridae. The virus can survive for a prolonged period of time in dry condition i.e scabs. It agglutinates RBCs and can be cultured in chorio-allantoic membrane of the developing chicken embryo. Here it produces typical pock like lesions. It also can be grown in chicken embryo fibroblast cell culture. The inoculation of ducks with fowl pox virus produces no lesions while inoculation of chickens with duck pox virus produces mild pox infection. Ducks immunized with fowl pox vaccine are susceptible to duck pox virus infection.

Epidemiology

It is worldwide in prevalence. Birds of all ages, sexes and breeds are susceptible. The virus has been isolated from 60 species of wild birds representing 20 families. Usually, it occurs as a sporadic disease in ducks but outbreaks have also reported.

Transmission

The pox disease spreads through contact and also by intermediate hosts like mosquitoes (Culex, Aedes), ticks, biting flies and lice which generally produces cutaneous lesions while aerosol infection causes diphtheritic form.

Pathogenesis

All the different stages of typical pox lesions may occur but commonly there will be hyperplasia of the epithelial cells of the skin and later on scab like lesions appearing like warts.

Clinical findings

The pox virus infections generally occur in three forms as in fowl fox

1. *Cutaneous form*: Wart like lesions is seen on the combs, wattles, eyelids, corner of beak and later on legs, feet and vent.
2. *Oculo-nasal form*: Lesions are seen in the eye and nasal cavity with coryza like signs.
3. *Diptheritic or oral form*: In this form nodular type of lesions are seen on the side of tongue, palate, epiglottis and also infra-orbital sinus, pharynx, larynx, oesophagus. The nodules coalesce together to form a diptheritic membrane. These lesions come in the way of ingestion of water and feed and also respiration. In this form majority of bird died due to asphyxia.

Diagnosis

The diagnosis of disease may be easily done based on typical signs and lesions.

By demonstration of inclusion bodies- the virus produces intra-cytoplasmic inclusion bodies called *Bollinger bodies* which are 2-3 in diameter and contains small granules called *borrel granules*. These can be demonstrated in the epithelial cells from the lesions. Scabs can be sent to laboratory.

Isolation of virus: The scab can be submitted. Here also by using CAM method of the chicken embryos the pock lesions on the CAM develops and is confirmed by HA and HI tests.

Serological tests: HIT, AGPT, FAT, ELISA, VNT.

Treatment

There is no specific treatment for fowl pox as it is viral disease.

Control

Isolation of affected fowls and general hygienic measures.

Vaccination: Fowl pox vaccine may give protection but no scientific evidence is available.

Fowl pox vaccine, live chick embryo virus (freeze dried): It is modified living virus vaccine (MLV) prepared from CAM of the chicken embryo and used in fowls but not in pigeons.

100 dose vaccine is available.

Mode of administration: The tip of medium sized sewing needle at the eye end is broken and rubbed on the stone to make it smooth. Hold the wing of the bird, dip the needle in the vaccine and make 2 punctures in the wing. This is called wing web puncture method. Examine the vaccinated bird after 7 days for take.

Pigeon pox vaccine: This vaccine can be used to protect the birds (fowls, pigeons) of all age group and also adult birds in the face of an outbreak. It is available in 100 and 500 doses with diluents

Mode of administration: Remove few feathers from one side of the thigh of the bird. Dip the Johnsons ear bud or glass rod with the cotton swab in the vaccine and paint the lesion where the feathers have been removed.

Fowl pox B-M strain (Bio-Med): 100 and 500 doses available. It is a live attenuated vaccine. The vaccine is reconstituted and 0.2 ml is injected i/m or s/c in the thigh region.

First Dose: 14-15 weeks

Second Dose: 16-18 weeks

Fowl pox vaccine (live) (BAIF): 200 and 500 doses with diluents. It is a modified fowl pox virus vaccine. Administered using wing web method in 6-8 weeks old chickens and then every year it is repeated.

References

Chen, Y.P., Yu, C.F. and Shih, Y.H. (2022). Duck Diseases and Disease Management. In Duck Production and Management Strategies (pp. 549-579). Springer, Singapore.

Dhama, K., Kumar, N., Saminathan, M., Tiwari, R., Karthik, K., Kumar, A., Palanivelu, M., Shabbir, M.Z., Malik, Y.Z. and Singh, R.K. (2014). Epiedmiology of Duck Viral Enteritis. DOI: 10.2478/bvip-2014-0078

Eldin, W. F. S. and Reda, L.M. (2016). Epidemiological prevalence of Pasteurellamultocida in ducks. Japanese Journal of Veterinary Research. 64(2)251-255.

Kozdruń, W., Czekaj, H. and Lorek, M. Outbreak of duck viral hepatitis in duckling flocks in Poland. Bull Vet InstPulawy. 58:513-515.

Pantin-Jackwood MJ, Swayne DE. (2009). Pathogenesis and pathobiology of avian influenza virus infection in birds. Rev Sci Tech., 28(1):113-36. PMID: 19618622.

Tuula Hollmén, J. Christian Franson, Douglas E. Docherty, Mikael Kilpi, Martti Hario, Lynn H. Creekmore, Margaret R. Petersen, (2000). Infectious Bursal Disease Virus Antibodies in Eider Ducks and Herring Gulls, The Condor, Volume 102, Issue 3, Pages 688–691, https://doi.org/10.1093/condor/102.3.688

Vegad, J. L. and Katiyar, A. K. (2005). A Text Book of Veterinary Special Pathology. Infectious diseases of livestock and poultry. IBDC, Lucknow.

9

Protozoan Diseases of Ducks

Protozoa are single celled eukaryotes which are either parasitic or free living belonged to family apicomplexa. These protozoan affects the different birds like chickens, turkey, ducks, pigeons, game birds and also various pet birds. The infection caused by protozoan diseases may affect one system or more than one system of the body depending on the causative agents involved. The common protozoan diseases like leukocytozonosis, chochlosomiasis, cryptosporidiosis, coccidiosis, histoplasmosis causes infection in the ducks. The protozoan diseases cause severe economic loss to the poultry industry due to death of birds, expenditure on the treatment and prevention of disease and loss of egg and meat production.

Leukocytozoonosis

It is a vector borne blood protozoan disease of duck primarily caused by *Leucocytozoon simondi* and commonly characterized by anaemia, diarrhoea and nervous signs.

Etiology

Leucocytozoon belongs to phylum Apicomplexa and the species of this genus uses black flies (*Simulium*) or biting midges as definitive host and birds as intermediate host. The Leukocytozoon infects the various captive and free-living species of avian but in water fowl it is caused by *Leucocytozoon simondi.*

Epidemiology

In ducks, outbreak has reported from North America, Asia and Europe. It causes mostly sub clinical infections but occasionally causes clinical and fatal infections. Mortality among birds fluctuates significantly with the strain of parasite, species, degree of exposure, age, immune status, and other factors. The ducklings are mostly affected with acute form while adults are affected with sub-acute or chronic form.

Transmission

The arthropod vectors like black flies (*S. anatinum* and *S. rugglesi*) acts as definitive host and transmission of leucocytozoonosis increases with increase in their population. Recovered birds usually acts as a carrier and source of infections to young birds.

Pathogenesis

The parasites enter the blood of bird as sporozoites through the bite of blood sucking black fly. The sporozoites invade the host cell in liver and undergoes asexual reproduction and produces numerous merozoites. The merozoites infects erythrocytes, leucocytes, macrophages or endothelial cells and develop into megaloschizonts. In erythrocytes and leukocytes merozoites develop into gametocytes. These gametocytes are taken by blood sucking fly while biting the host and mature as macrogametocytes (female) with red staining nuclei and microgametocytes (male) with pale staining diffuse nuclei. These two fuses together form ookinete and penetrate the intestinal wall and mature as oocyst and after several days sporozoites are released to salivary gland of fly. The clinical signs and mortality are due to anemia associated with anti-erythrocytic factors produced by the parasite. The large gametocytes block pulmonary capillaries or parasites invading the endothelium of vessels in tissues like brain, heart, etc where it forms megaloschizonts that occlude vessels and result in multifocal necrosis.

The parasitemia mostly increases with rise of arthropod vectors number in spring season. The recovered ducks show relapse of infection of *L. simondi* due to increased level of prolactin when light cycle is manipulated to increase egg production.

Clinical signs

The clinical signs include loss of appetite, anaemia, diarrhoea with green droppings, listlessness, rapid breathing, weakness, and occasionally death within 24 hours in ducklings. In adult ducks signs of disease usually develop gradually with milder signs and most of the affected birds die in a few days. The adult ducks may have continuous cough, tracheal rales, loss of vigor, reduced mating and birds often die when under stress. The mortality rate in ducking may be upto 70% and low in adult ducks.

Post mortem findings

The peritoneal, perirenal, and subdural hemorrhages, splenomegaly, hepatomegaly present in severe cases. Histologically megaloschizont development is present in the spleen, liver, heart, and other organs.

Diagnosis

The diagnosis is based on the clinical signs of anaemia, leukocytosis, tachypnea, anorexia, diarrhoea with green droppings and CNS signs in ducklings, *In blood smear Leucocytozoon* is identified by large gametocytes that lack pigment and present in distorted RBC or WBC. The gametocytes may be elongated with long tapering extremities, whereas others are round. Serology tests and PCR tests have been developed for diagnosis of leukocytozoonosis.

Treatment

Treatment is not much effective but primaquine 0.75-1 mg/kg PO once, used in conjunction with chloroquine (25 mg/kg PO at 0h, then 15 mg/kg at 12,24, and 48h) and Pyrimethamine Given orally (0.5 mg/kg PO q12h x 14-28 days) or in feed (1 mg/kg feed for 28 days), Supplement with folic acid has shown promising effects.

Cochlosomiasis

It is a disease of duck and turkey caused by *Cochlosoma anatis* characterized by gastrointestinal distress.

Etiology

It is caused by *Cochlosoma anatis* which is 6–12 mcm long and 4–7 mcm wide, with a characteristic adhesive disc on the anteroventral surface of its pyriform body. It moves in a jerking motion. This protozoan has a single nucleus and uses flagella for movement. Kotlán described first about the Cochlosoma in 1923 to include *C. anatis*, a flagellate present in the intestines of young European domestic ducks (Anas platyrhynchos) infected with coccidiosis. *Cochlosoma rostratum* later considered as *C. anatis* was identified in North American domestic ducks by Kimura in 1934.

Epidemiology

It infects duck, turkey, geese and wild birds. Wild birds, small rodents, and multi-aged flocks have been identified as carriers of *C anatis.*

Transmission

Transmission commonly takes place through faeco-oral route. Lateral transmission has been observed with turkeys, but direct contact of the birds was necessary for infection. PCR has detected *C. anatis* on house flies, but no studies have demonstrated them as carrying live trophozoites.

Pathogenesis

The exact mechanism of pathogenesis is not known. The coinfection of viruses, bacteria and other protozoans with *C anatis* may causes gastrointestinal distress but alone infection of *C. anatis* does not produce any clinical signs. The *C anatis* attaches to intestinal mucosa without any visual changes in the intestine under light microscopy. The multiplication of *C. anatis* takes place by longitudinal binary fission and pseudocyst act as a source of infection in faeco-oral route.

Clinical signs

The common clinical manifestation associated with this disease in duckings, wild and domestic turkey poults are runting and catarrhal enteritis. The cochlosoma may be present as main pathogen or also in combination with Coccidiosis, Salmonella and Hexamita.

Diagnosis

The light microscopy and PCR are useful in the diagnosis of disease from intestinal scrapping and faeces.

Differential Diagnosis

It may be differentiated with diseases of smilikar clinical signs like salmonellosis, pasteurellosis, duck plaque, duck parvo virus infection etc.

Treatment and Prevention

The strict biosecurity measures to prevents the entry of rodents and wild birds is needed to prevent the contamination of flocks. The Nitrcimidazole and nitarsone have been proven as successful treatments for chochlodomiasis.

Coccidiosis

Coccidiosis is a parasitic disease of intestinal tract of bird, livestocks and human characterized by haemorrhagic enteririts , diarrhoea emaciation, weight loss, decreased production and even death.

Etiology

Coccidiosis in wild and farmed duck caused by Eimeria, Isospora, Tyzzeria, and Wenyonella genera and 13 species of coccidia have been reported in ducks. Both domestic and wild ducks are commonly infected with coccidian. Coccidiosis in birds and animals are mostly host specific. The young or immunecompromised animals may have severe clinical signs and death while most of the infected birds or animals are asymptomatic.

Epidemiology

Coccidiosis is one of the most common and economically important diseases of ducks. Coccidiosis in ducks has been reported from several countries like

United States, Denmark, England, Japan, India, Canada, Iceland and China. Ducklings below 7 weeks of age reported high mortality as they are most severely affected with coccidiosis.

Transmission

Transmission of coccidiosis in ducks is caused by faeco-oral route. The infection occurs by ingestion of sporulated oocysts. The un-sporulated oocysts are passed out in the faeces, which under favourable environmental condition sporulate and become infective. The oocysts can also be transmitted mechanically through carriers like farm equipment, clothings, insects and other animals.

Pathogenesis

The sporulated oocysts enters into the intestine through ingestion. The small intestines of ducks infected with *Tyzzeria perniciosa* are often distended and filled with blood and caseous exudate while *T. perniciosa* causes mortality upto 30%. The recovered ducks are usually associated with slow weight gain. Sloughing of the intestinal wall in long sheets may also be seen and the coccidia may invade very deep to the muscular layers of the intestinal wall.

Clinical signs

Severe enteritis and haemorrhagic diarrhoea is seen with the most pathological strains of the disease along with mucoid discharge. Weight loss, reduced appetite and depression are other common signs. *T. perniciosa* causes ballooning of the entire small intestine with muco-hemorrhagic or caseous material.

Necropsy findings

Macroscopically extensive haemorrhages in the intestine, sloughing of intestinal mucosa and microscopically presence of few or no oocysts, large number of merozoites in intestinal sloughing.

Diagnosis

- History and clinical signs are useful in tentative diagnosis of coccidiosis in ducks.
- Detection of duck coccidia oocysts in feces or ureteral contents confirms diagnosis.
- Post mortem examination of the presence of caseous core lesions in the caecum and exuviating of the bowel walls are helpful in diagnosis.
- Histopathological studies demonstrate different developmental stage on staining.

- Haematological and molecular approaches such as isoenzyme analysis, SDS-PAGE, pulse field gel electrophoresis, restriction enzyme digestion and southern blot analysis and the most recent PCR including RAPD-PCR etc.

Differential Diagnosis

The coccidiosis in ducks should be differentiated from salmonellosis, cryptosporidiosis, duck viral hepatitis, colibacillosis etc.

Treatment

The drugs used for treatment of clinical coccidiosis in chicken may be useful in the treatment of coccidiosis in ducks. The medicines are usually given in drinking water except tetracycline, which is usually administered in feed. The coccidiosis may be prevented by using 30 gm of Amprolium soluble (20%) powder/50 lit of drinking water for 5-7 days. The mild infection may be treated by using 25 gm of amprolium in 30 liter of drinking water and in severe infection 60 gm per 30 liter of drinking water for 5-7 days. The combination of amprolium (240ppm) and sulphaquinocaline (180ppm) for 3-6 days and amprolium (125ppm) and ethopabate (8 ppm) for 5-7 days are effective against coccidiosis. Sulphadimethoxine (0.05%) for 6 days, sulphamethazine (0.1%) for 2 days, toltrazuril (25-75 ppm) for 2 days, pyrimethazine (0.1%) and sulphaquinoxoline (14 ppm) combination for 3 days repeated again for 3 days after an interval of 2 days. Chlortetracycline (0.022%) with calcium (0.8%) for upto 3 weeks and Oxytetracycline (0.022%) with calcium (0.18-0.55%) for 5 days is also effective

Prevention and Control

The affected ducks should be identified and isolated from the healthy birds. The prevention of coccidiosis is usually done by administration of any one drug mentioned under treatment either in feed or drinking water to day old chicks and continued for prolonged period of time. Good hygiene measures should be followed and overcrowding among ducks should be avoided as much as possible. Contaminated feeder and waterer should be avoided. The bedding and surrounding should be sterilized by using 1.25% sodium hypochlorite or 0.5% cresol or phenol or by fumigation with formaldehyde. Before stocking the new batch thorough scrubbing with hot detergent like 10% ammonia for 45 min or methy bromide @ 5 mg/lit for 20 hours, should be done. To prevent the resistance, the anti-coccidial agents to be used for chemoprophylaxis should be rotated after every 4-6 months. A change from floor to cages greatly reduces the exposure of coccidiosis. Supplementation of Vitamin K, A, C or E exerts beneficial effects due to decrease clotting time, antioxidant, membrane stabilizing and immunomodulating properties.

Cryptosporidiosis

Cryptosporidiosis is a zoonotic, protozoal disease caused by genus Cryptosporidia and characterized by respiratory and gastrointestinal disorder in ducks.

Etiology

Cryptosporidiosis in ducks is commonly caused by *C. baleyi* and *C. meleagridis*. It is not host specific and can affect various species of animals.

Epidemiology

The Cryptosporidiosis is naturally prevalent in birds like quail, pheasants, peafowl, waterfowl, chickens, turkeys, finches and psittacines. It is poorly host specific and can affect different species of animals including human being. Experimentally it has been observed that ducks are more resistant respiratory cryptosporidiosis caused by *C. baileyi* than are chickens and turkeys.

Transmission

The inhalation or ingestion of oocysts passed in the droppings of infected birds are the main source of infection to susceptible birds. The oocysts are very resistant in the environment and carried between flocks by direct or indirect mode like equipment, feeding and watering troughs etc.

Pathogenesis

The pathogenesis of cryptosporidiosis is not well known and the cause of profuse diarrhoea in affected birds is considered due to enterotoxin production but scientifically it is not proven. The multiplication of oocysts after entry into the intestine causes production of merozoites which is responsible for degenerative changes and atrophy of villi in large intestine. The immense damage to microvilli causes secretion of water and electrolyte into intestine which is showed by watery diarrhoea. The immunity of the birds generally determines the course of cryptosporidiosis in host.

Clinical signs

Cryptosporidium is generally present in the sinuses, trachea, bronchi, cloaca, and bursa of chicken, turkey nad ducks which lead to coughing, gasping, airsacculitis, and sometimes death. The diarrhoea and dehydration are the most common clinical signs reported among the affected ducks. The clinical signs of disease may be present in affected birds for several weeks.

Necropsy findings

Diagnosis

On microscopic examination the small oocysts (5mcm) present in the tissue scrapings or histologic examination of tissues from the bursa, cloaca, and trachea or by examination of faecal sample by floatation technique. Concentration of intestinal scrapings using saturated sugar solution and examination. The phase-contrast or interference-contrast microscopy may improve visualization of oocysts.

Differential Diagnosis

Cryptosporidiosis in ducks may be differentiate with Cochlosomiasis, Coccidiosis, Duck viral enteritis, Pasteurellosis etc.

Treatment

The effective treatment for cryptosporidiosis in ducks is not available but many ducks may recover on their own. The all known anticoccidial drugs are ineffective against cryptosporidiosis in ducks.

Prevention and Control

The suitable control measures for the control of cryptosporidiosis infections in ducks are lacking and is only based on good hygiene, sanitation and biosecurity measures. The cryptosporidia spp are extremely resistant to most of the chemical disinfectant and steam cleaning may inactivate the oocysts above about 65^{0}C. The bird died of cryptosporidiosis should be incinerated.

Avian Trichomoniasis

Trichomoniasis is a highly contagious protozoan disease among birds caused by tetra *Trichomonas anati* and characterized by respiratory and intestinal form in ducks.

Aetiology

It is caused by *Trichomonas gallinae* in domestic pigeons and birds. It also occurs in chicken, turkey, ducks, dove and sparrow. The organisms are pyriform in shape, having 4 anterior flagella. The undulating membrane does not reach upto the posterior end of the body. The free trailing flagellum is absent. In ducks the causative agent is morphologically identified as tetra *Trichomonas anati.*

In pigeon disease is transmitted from adults to squabs through pigeon milk. Hawks and golden eagle get the infection by eating infected pigeons while chicken, turkey etc get it by drinking contaminated water. The adult birds remain infected for a year or more and are a constant source of infection for their young once.

Clinical findings

In the first outbreak, main clinical signs were. Histological lesions were confined to the upper respiratory tract and lower small intestine and consisted of mucofibrino-purulent sinusitis and catarrhal rhinitis, tracheitis and enteritis. The protozoa appeared frequently in the infraorbital sinuses, the respiratory region of the nose, and the lower small intestine, but rarely in the trachea. In the second outbreak, the lesions were limited to the lower small intestine with catarrhal enteritis in adult ducks clinically showing profuse diarrhoea and low mortality.

The adult ducks usually harbor symptomless infection whereas young birds suffer severely. The affected birds lose weight and may fall if forced to move. In respiratory form bilateral swelling of infraorbital sinuses, sneezing, high mortality present in young ducks. In intestinal form lesions are limited to small intestine and characterized with catarrhal enteritis in adult ducks showing profuse diarrhoea and low mortality. The protozoa appeared frequently in the infraorbital sinuses, the respiratory region of the nose, and the lower small intestine, but rarely in the trachea.

Necropsy findings

In ducks, histological lesions were confined to the upper respiratory tract and lower small intestine and consisted of mucofibrino-purulent sinusitis and catarrhal rhinitis, tracheitis and enteritis.

Diagnosis

Based on history and clinical signs.

Culture: The organism can be readily cultured on a variety of media like glucose-broth-serum medium or trypticase-yeast extract-maltose-cysteine-serum medium.

Differential Diagnosis

Thrush: Fungus can be seen in smears and sections and can be cultured in special media.

Fowl pox: Nodular lesions frequently occur on unfeathered skin.

Vitamin A deficiency: Keratinisation of the epithelial cells of the olfactory, respiratory, upper gastro-intestinal and urinary tracts. White or grayish white urate deposits can be seen in kidneys, ureters and other organs.

Treatment

Antiprotozoal drugs like dimetridazole, metronidazole, copper sulfate, quaternary ammonia, carnidazole, 2-amino-5-nitrothiazole and amino-nitrothiazole are effective against trichomoniasis in birds. Carnidazole in a single dose and metronidazole can be used for 2-10 days via oral application

Prevention and Control

Prevention and control involve removal of the source of infective organisms and treatment of infected ducks. Source removal often requires the destruction of chronically infected birds and protection of water sources from wild birds. Oral antiprozoan drugs are useful in minimizing the infection in birds. The new ducks only introduce in the flock after 30 days of quarantine.

Sarcocystosis (Rice Bread Disease)

Sarcocystosis is an infection of mammal, reptiles and birds caused by parotozoa of the genus Sarcocystis and characterized by torticollis, trembling, paralysis in ducks.

Etiology

The genus Sarcocystis includes more than 200 known species but ducks are affected by *S. horvathi* and *S. wenzeli*, which are present in definitive host dogs and cats. The sarcocystis oocysts (eggs) excreted in the faeces of dog and cat which acts as sources of infection to ducks through ingestion.

Epidemiology

Incidence

Sarcocystosis is worldwide in distribution. Dogs, cats and opossum acts as definitive host and birds act as intermediate host. It may infect the all mammals, reptiles and birds.

Transmission

Parasites live in definitive host for reproduction and produces oocysts which may remain infective in the environment for months. After ingestion, oocysts hatch into merozoites which invade the duck's muscle tissue.

Pathogenesis

The sporocysts ingestion by a suitable intermediate host causes release of sporozoites and initiate development of schizonts occurs in vascular endothelia of mesenteric arterioles and lymph nodes. The various organs produce second generation of endothelial schizonts in their capillaries. The merozoites produced from these schizonts enter into the muscle fibers and develop into the typical sarcocysts. The sporocyst contains only a few metrocytes (rounded cells), which give rise to the banana-shaped infective bradyzoites found in mature cysts after 2 to 3 months of infection.

Clinical signs

Waterfowl and carnivore hosts that are infected with sarcocysts usually appear healthy. When butchering infected ducks, cysts may be observed in the breast muscle. The cysts appear like grains of rice or whitish streaks running in the direction of the muscle fibers, gave the name as rice bread disease. The common clinical signs of torticollis, depression, polyuria, trembling and paralysis are present in ducks.

Post mortem findings

The gross examination of cysts appears like grains of rice or whitish streaks running in the direction of the muscle fibers specially in brisket muscle. The microscopic examination of muscle shows presence of sarcocysts along with myositis, myonecrosis, perivascular and interstitial inflammation, vasculitis, and eosinophilic myositis.

Diagnosis

The biopsy of infected muscle and its staining with haematoxylin and eosin are useful in definitive diagnosis of sarcocysts. The microscopic examination along with sarcocysts also shows myositis, myonecrosis, perivascular and interstitial inflammation, vasculitis, and eosinophilic myositis. The PAS stain is also helpful with variable uptake of stain. The faecal examination also revealed the presence of oocysts under microscope.

Treatment

The treatment against sarcocystosis is not much effective. The drugs like pyrimithamine0.25 to 0.5 mg/kg b wt orally twice daily for one month and Trimethoprime-sulphadiazine combination 60 mg/kg b wt., p.o or s/c twice daily for 3 days then 2 days off then again for 3 days has shown promising results.

Prevention and Control

There is no effective treatment against chronic intracellular sarcocysts as most species have a prey-predator life cycle. The main control strategies are to prevent ingestion of prey carcasses or raw tissues by omnivorous or carnivorous animals and to reduce grass and water contamination with their feces to minimize the oocysts exposure to birds. Supplies of grain and feed should not come in contact with dogs and cats.

Haemosporidiosis (Avian Malaria)

Avian Malaria is a parasitic disease of ducks caused by blood protozoa *Plasmodium* spp., and haemoproteus spp and characterized by anorexia, haemolytic anaemia, haemoglobinuria and high mortality.

Etiology

Avian malaria is a parasitic disease of birds, caused by parasite species belonging to the genera *Plasmodium* and *Haemoproteus* and transmitted by a dipteran vector including mosquitoes in *Plasmodium* parasites and biting midges for *Hemoproteus*. Schizogony occurs in the RBC and, therefore, blood-to-blood transfer without the intermediate host can result in infection. *P. gallinaceum*, *P. juxtanucleare* and *P. durae* may cause up to 90% mortality in poultry.

Epidemiology

The various species of poultry including ducks, geese, swans and other waterfowl are extremely susceptible to infection. In outbreaks upto 75 percent of wild waterfowl species are reported to be infected with hematozoa parasites. These parasites are transmitted to ducks through various insect-vectors like black flies (*Simulium* spp), louse flies (*Ornithomyia* spp), biting midges (*Culicoides* spp), and mosquitoes (*Culex, Aedes* spp). These vectors mostly feed on the exposed flesh around the eyes, the beak and on the legs and feet of the bird while many biting flies can crawl beneath the duck's feathers to reach the skin surface. The three genera most commonly reported in waterfowl include Leucocytozoon, Ducks with existing parasitic infections are more at risk of a secondary infection resulting from immune-suppression.

Pathogenesis

The biting of infected mosquitoes causes, RBC of birds to be infected and after few days acute phase of infection occurs in which parasite number rapidly increases to reach a peak parasitemia. The rapid multiplication of asexual stages in blood causes burst of infected RBC leading to anemic crisis and anoxia which is characterized by rapid loss of body mass. Infection is usually controlled by immune response involving a series of immune effectors and inflammatory cytokines and also by clearance of RBC by spleen. After activation of immune response birds enter a chronic phase of infection which is characterized by low level of parasitaemia for years.

Clinical signs

The disease is clinically characterized by weak, depression and anorexia, abdominal protrusion due to splenomegaly, haemolytic anaemia and haemoglobinurira. The central nervous signs may be present and coma and death may occur quickly in high parasitaemia. Some birds, especially passerines, do not become ill and play an important role as asymptomatic carriers of the parasite.

Diagnosis

Blood smear examination using Wright's stain is a sensitive method to detect *Plasmodium* intra-erythrocytic trophozoites, schizonts and gametocytes. The trophozoite appears like "signet ring" like which is small round to oval structure with a large vacuole that forces the erythrocyte nucleus to one pole. Schizonts are round to oval inclusions in the red cells containing darkly-stained merozoites. The schizonts can be detected in capillaries of brain, lung, liver, and spleen. by using impression smears.PCR is also useful in diagnose *Plasmodium*.

Treatment

The anti-protozoal drugs like chloroquine phosphate potentiated with primaquine in drinking water is useful. Sulfonamides combined with trime-thoprim, pyrimethamine, and chlorguanil. are also helpful.

Prevention and Control

The success of management strategies for avian malaria depends primarily on controlling mosquitoes that carry *Plasmodium*. It may be achieved by the elimination of standing-water catchments that attract breeding mosquitoes and finding the ways to develop genetic resistance in sensitive species.

References

Callait-Cardinal MP, Chauve C, Reynaud MC, Alogninouwa T, Zenner L. Infectivity of Histomonasmeleagridis in ducks. Avian Pathol. 2006 Apr;35(2):109-16. doi: 10.1080/03079450600597626 PMID: 16595302.

Chapman HD (2014). Milestones in avian coccidiosis research: A review. Poultry Science 93: 501-511.

Franssen FFJ and Lumeij JT (1992). In vitro nitroimidazole resistance of Trichomonas gallinae and successful therapy with an increased dosage of ronidazole in racing pigeons (*Columba livia domestica*). Journal of Veterinary Pharmacology and Therapeutics, 15(4):409-415; 20

Kalifa MM, Nassar AM, Nisreen EM & Abdel-Wahab AM (2016). Cryptosporidium species in ducks: parasitological, serological and molecular studies in Egypt. International Journal of Advanced Research in Biological Sciences 3: 23-31.

Kuhn, Ryan C et al. (2002). "Occurrence of Cryptosporidium and Giardia in wild ducks along the Rio Grande River valley in southern New Mexico." Applied and Environmental Microbiology, 68,1: 161-5. doi:10.1128/AEM.68.1.161-165.2002

Laatamna AE, Holubová N, Sak B &Kvác M (2017). Cryptosporidium meleagridisand *C. baileyi* (Apicomplexa) in domestic and wild birds in Algeria. Folia Parasitologica, 64: 1-7.

Lindsay, David S., et al. (1989). "Experimental Infections in Domestic Ducks with Cryptosporidium Baileyi Isolated from Chickens." Avian Diseases, 33,(1): 69–73. JSTOR, https://doi.org/10.2307/1591069.Accessed 27 May 2022.

Mason, R. W. (1986). "Conjunctival Cryptosporidiosis in a Duck." Avian Diseases 30, no. 3: 598-600.

McDougald LR & Fitz-Coy SH (2008). "Coccidiosis in Ducks" in Saif YM (ed.) Diseases of Poultry. Blackwell Publishing, Iowa, USA, pp. 1083-1084.

Pecka, Z., Nohynkova, E., and Kulda, J. 1996: Ultrastructure of Cochlosoma anatis Kotlan, 1923 and taxonomic position of the family Cochlosomatidae (Parabasala: *Trichomonadida*). Eur. J. Protistol. 32: 190-201. doi: 10.1016/S0932-4739(96)80019-8

Ricklefs, R. E.; Fallon, S. M. (2002). "Diversification and host switching in avian malaria parasites". Proceedings of the Royal Society of London B: Biological Sciences. 269 (1494): 885–892. doi:10.1098/rspb.2001.1940. ISSN 0962-8452. PMC 1690983. PMID 12028770

Rogers, K. (2019, March 18). avian malaria. Encyclopedia Britannica. https://www.britannica.com/science/avian-malaria.

Sparks H, Nair G, Castellanos-Gonzalez A and White AC Jr. (2015). Treatment of Cryptosporidium: What We Know, Gaps, and the Way Forward. Curr Trop Med Rep. 2(3):181-187.

Travis, B.V. 1938: A synopsis of the flagellate Genus Cochlosoma Kotlan with the dexcription of two new species. J. Parasitol. 24: 343-351. doi: 10.2307/3272444.

Tsai SS, Chang TC, Kuo M and Itakura C (1997). Respiratory and intestinal trichomoniasis in mule ducks. Avian Pathol. 1997;26(3):651-6. doi: 10.1080/03079459708419241. PMID: 18483934.

Watkins, R.A., O'Dell, W.D., and Pinter, A.J. 1989: Redescription of flagellar arrangement in the duck intestinal flagellate, Cochlosoma anatis and description of a new species, Cochlosoma soricis N. Sp. From Shrews. J. Protozool. 36(6): 527-532.

Williams, R.B. 2013: Nomenclatural and bibliographical notes on new taxa of protozoan parasites described by Ernest Edward Tyzzer (1875–1965). Zoological Bibliography. 2(4): 131-142.

Williams RB (2005) Avian Malaria: clinical and chemical pathology of Plasmodium gallinaceum in the domesticated fowl Gallus gallus Avian Pathology 34(1), 29-47.

Wu H-L (2016). Prevalence of Wenyonella philiplevinei infection in Linwu ducks in Linwu county, subtropical China. Tropical Animal Health and Production 48: 659-662.

10

Fungal Diseases of Ducks

Fungus is member of group of eukaryotic organisms that includes yeasts and molds. The fungi are heterotrophs and they acquire their food by absorbing dissolved molecules by secreting digestive enzyme in the environment. It is present in common place in the environment and some are normal inhabitants of the skin, gastrointestinal tract and other mucous membrane surfaces. Generally if birds immunity is intact and fully operational then it will overcome the fungal infection in most situations, In case of compromised immune system it will cause development of serious infections. Paramount to properly managing fungal infections in avian species is the ability to recognize infection early in the course of disease, to administer appropriate antifungal medications for the location and severity of infection, and to continually assess a patient's response to therapy.

Avian candidiasis

Avian candidiasis is mycosis of digestive tract of chick, turkey, geese, pigeon, guinea fowl and other birds which occur secondary in susceptible ducks affected to other diseases. It generally occurs secondary to other diseases in duck.

Etiology

Candidiasis in duck is primarily caused by *Candida albicans* which is a yeast-like single celled opportunistic pathogen and normal inhabitant of the crop in healthy birds. It generally occurs in ducks with stress, immunocompromised, beak abnormalities, impacted food or parasitic loads, tongue injuries, receiving prolonged antibiotic therapy or affected by a primary disease are susceptible for secondary infection of candidiasis.

Epidemiology

The disease occurs frequently sporadically in immunocompromised or diseased ducks as secondary infection. It is of economic importance particularly in the turkey farming and even 20% or more mortality is observed in young turkeys. It is thought that the disease generally develops after the prolonged use of antibiotics or after deficiency of vitamin A, stress, delayed crop emptying, mal nutrition etc. Generalized candidiasis infection reported in Muscovy duck disease in Muscovy ducks and in a Muscovy duck/domestic duck hybrid. Younger and older ducks are more susceptible for candidiasis infections.

Pathogenesis

Candida infections of the skin and superficial mucosal sites are the outcome of an interaction between fungal virulence and host defenses. Epidermal proliferation and T-lymphocyte immune responses are expressed by the host to combat fungal attack, but inflammatory responses and nonspecific inhibitors also possibly play a role. *Candida albicans* can express at least three types of surface adhesion molecules to colonize epithelial surfaces, along with an aspartyl proteinase enzyme which is able to facilitate initial penetration of keratinized cells. Deeper penetration of keratinized epithelia is assisted by hypha formation, and *C. albicans* hyphae may use contact sensing (thigmotropism) as a guiding mechanism. Pathogenesis requires differential expression of virulence factors at each new stage of the process.

Clinical findings

The duck oral cavity may show white to cream, cheesy patches or plaques in crop, tongue, mouth, and esophagus tissue. The lesions may give the impression as necrotic patches which may be easily peeled off from the eroded mucosal surface. The crop may show white curd-like plaques and reddening of the nearby tissue. The infected ducks may seem 'yeasty or sour-like' breath, lethargic, dehydrated, little to no appetite, mild conjunctivitis and loss of condition. The ducks infected with candidiasis may have concurrent infection of other diseases.

Necropsy findings

There is thickening of mucosa with whitish, circular, raised ulcers formation. In acute cases, these lesions are greyish white, loosely adhere to the underlying surface and rather resemble with curdled milk.

In chronic cases crop wall is thickened and membrane is covered by corrugated mass of piled up yellowish white necrotic materials resembling turkey towels. The mouth and oesophagus may show ulcerative patches. When the proventriculus is involved, it is swollen, serosa has a glossy appearance and mucosa is haemorrhagic and may covered with catarrhal or necrotic exudates.

Diagnosis

Clinical symptoms are not specific, so give very little idea about the disease.

Direct microscopic examination: Presence of yeast cell and pseudo-hyphae is of diagnostic importance.

Culture examination and physiological character: *C. albican* ferment maltose and glucose, sometimes sucrose but never lactose and form chlamydospores on corn meal agar and germ tubes in serum

Treatment

Administration of nystatin @ 70-125 mg/kg feed or in drinking water helps in preventing the further spread of the disease and 20 gm of mycostatin/tonn of feed completely destroys Candida from crop of birds.

Haymicin is effective against *C. albicans* and can be used for local application or given orally @ 10 ml suspension in drinking water.

Copper sulphate at 1:2000 dilutions in the drinking water is effective both as control and prophylactic measure against in the poultry.

Cleanliness, proper management, adequate vitamin A supplement and judicious use of antibiotics are essential for the prevention of the disease.

Prevention

The clean environment, balanced nutrition, minimizing the any causes of stress, and stopping contact with sick birds, decreases the chances of candidiasis in ducks.

Ducks or duckling on prolonged antibiotic treatment should be supplemented with antifungal agents like nystatin or itraconazole to avoid the occurrence of candidiasis. These anti-fungal agents may be added in the had rearing formula of the ducklings.

Aspergilosis (Fungal Pneumonia, Mycosis Aspergillosis)

It is a common, non-contagious fungal infection of ducks caused by Aspergillus spp. and commonly characterized by respiratory tract infections in ducks.

Etiology

Aspergillosis is most commonly caused by *A. fumigatus* among the various species isolated from clinically infected ducks. Aspergillus spp. are widespread, opportunistic in nature and healthy ducks are regularly exposed to fungal spores without causing any clinical signs. The ducks with compromised immune system are vulnerable to infections and usually result in concurrent infection.

Epidemiology

Incidence

Aspergillosis are worldwide in distribution and multiply rapidly with high humidity and warm temperatures (25°C). The all birds including domestic birds like chicken, duck, turkey etc and wild birds are susceptible to aspergillosis.

Transmission

The main mode of transmission of aspergillosis is inhalation of aspergillus spores (conidia) from contaminated feed, soil, faecal materials etc. The predisposing factors for aspergillosis are receiving antibiotics or steroids for longer duration, exposure to damp bedding, living in a warm, humid environment with poor air circulation, exposure to large accumulations of dust. The concurrent or chronic diseases, impairment of the immune system, overcrowded conditions, poor sanitary environment, moldy feed or regular exposure of moldy environment.

Pathogenesis

The large number of small, hydrophobic spores (conidia) enters into birds posterior thoracic and abdominal air sacs through nares. The air sacs epithelial surface is almost devoid of muco-ciliary transport mechanism and macrophages. Aspergillus spores of small size (2-3microns) enter into lungs and air sacs and germinate. Respiratory epithelial cells engulfed the conidia by endocytosis while some of the spore germinate externally and forming hyphae which penetrate and damage the cells by loss of cilia and detachment of cells. The endocytosis of conidia by endothelial cells causes disseminated mycosis through haematogenous route. The macrophage engulfs the conidia and kill it within the phagolysosome with reactive oxygen species (ROS) and phagolysosomal acidification. Aspergillosis commonly associated with immunosuppression in ducks.

Clinical signs

Clinical signs of aspergillosis vary extensively, depending on the various organs are affected. It can be either localized in particular organs or diffuse which results in a progressive, debilitating illness. Aspergillosis commonly affects the duck's upper and lower respiratory tract, although any organ systems can become infected in case of dissemination. Aspergillosis can be manifest as acute form when ducks are exposed to large number of conidia and chronic form, usually associated with immunosuppression. Acute form of aspergillosis generally develops within week of infection in young birds and causes high morbidity and mortality. The most commonly observed signs include depression, difficulty breathing, lethargy, loss of appetite, increased thirst, cyanosis, abdominal enlargement, and sometimes sudden death. The Chronic form is usually the most common form of aspergillosis in ducks and is most frequent in mature, adult ducks with history of antibiotics or corticosteroids treatment, previous disease, stressful event or chronic diseases. In this form clinical signs develop gradually and often non-specific like lethargy, anorexia, change in behavior, or weight loss in spite of good appetite. In case of air sacculitis due to infection of the air sacs with the fungus, clinical signs include increased respiratory effort, vocalization changes, tail-bobbing, open-mouthed breathing, and audible respiratory sounds.

Diagnosis

The diagnosis of aspergillosis in ducks, before death is curb some job and most of the time it is diagnosed after death based on postmortem findings of white caseous nodules in the lungs or air sacs of affected birds specially in chronic form. Definitive diagnosis is based on the isolation of Aspergillus species by culture or by the detection of the organism during histological examination

Differential stains such as Periodic acid-Schiff (PAS), Bauer's and Gridley's stains differentiate and easily identify the hyphae and mycelia. Grocott's and Gomori Methanamine Silver special stain is useful for the detection of fungal hyphae. Immunohistochemistry with monoclonal or polyclonal antibodies are also useful in detection of lesions in aspergillosis. Serological tests like immune-electrophoresis (CIE), agar gel immunodiffusion (AGI) and enzyme-linked immunosorbent assays (ELISA) are used for diagnosis.

Differential Diagnosis

The aspergillosis in ducks should be differentiated from diseases with similar clinical signs and lesions like chlaymydiophylosis, tuberculosis, neoplasm, vitamin A deficiency, pneumonia, candidiasis.

Treatment

The treatment of aspergillosis is very difficult and its outcome depends upon the location and extent of infection. In case of extensive infections in the tissue the prognosis is poor and only systemic drugs like itraconazole (5-10 mg twice a day, orally for 7-21 days), fluconazole (15 mg twice a day, orally for 7 days), clotrimazole (1%), miconazole (1%), ketoconazole (20-30 mg/kg b wt twice a day orally for 2-6 weeks) and amphotericin B (1 mg/kg b wt, iv, 3 to 4 times in day for 10-14 days) may be useful. The best treatment in granulomatous lesions are debridement and topical treatment in conjunction with a systemic therapy.

Prevention and Control

The reduction of predisposing immunosuppressive factors like malnutrition and stress minimizes the occurrence of aspergillosis as it is opportunistic pathogen. Standard of hygiene, nutrition and housing should be maintained. The mouldy and wet litter or feed should be avoided. The frequent disinfection of feeders, waterers and incubators should be done. Appropriate ventilation should be provided to maintain relative humidity so as to prevent wet litter. Environmental contamination should be control by spraying of fungistatic agents like nystatin, thiabendazole or copper sulphate (1 gram per 2 litre of water daily morning for 3 days). Anti-fungal drugs like itraconazole at 10mg/ kg once a day for 10 days orally have been used as prophylactic measures in birds with high risk to develop aspergillosis. To avoid the problem to future new borne the poultry breeder should disinfect eggs soon after being laid and gathered.

References

Ansson DS, Otman F, Bagge E, Lindgren Y, Etterlin PE, Eriksson H. Retrospective analysis of post-mortem findings in domestic ducks and geese from non-commercial flocks in Sweden, 2011-2020. Acta Vet Scand. 2021 Nov 24;63(1):47. doi: 10.1186/s13028-021-00614-x. PMID: 34819114; PMCID: PMC8613967.

Arné P, Thierry S, Wang D, Deville M, Le Loc'h G, Desoutter A, Féménia F, Nieguitsila A, Huang W, Chermette R and Guillot J (2011). Aspergillus fumigatus in Poultry. International Journal of Microbiology, Article ID 746356. Doi:10.1155/2011/746356. 14p.

Atasever A and Gümüşsoy K^S (2004). Pathological, clinical and mycological findings in experimental aspergillosis infections of starlings. Journal of Veterinary Medicine A -Physiology, Pathology, Clinical Medicine, 51(1): 19-22.

Barathidasan R, Singh SD, Saini M, Sharma AK and Dhama K (2013). The first case of angioinvasive pulmonary aspergillosis in a Himalayan Griffon Vulture (*Gyps himalayensis*). Avian Biology Research, 6(4): 302-306.

Barnett J, Booth P, Arrow M, Garcia-Rueda C and Irvine RM (2011). Spinal aspergillosis in pheasants. Veterinary Record, 169(17): 449-450

Leishangthem, G.D., Singh, N.D., Brar, R.S. and Bang, H.S (2015). Aspergillosis in Avian Species: A Review. Journal of Poultry Science and Technology 3(1):1-14.

Sadar, Miranda J., et al (2014). Mycotic keratitis in a khaki Campbell duck (*Anas platyrhynchos domesticus*) Journal of Avian Medicine and Surgery 28.4

Wang, S. and Suo, X. (2019).Coccidiosis in ducks (Anas sp.)" Coccidiosis in Livestock, Poultry, Companion Animals, and Humans. 1st Edn, CRC Press.

11

Parasitic Diseases of Ducks and Their Management

The domestic duck is an economically important domestic bird in rural areas. They are productive and are reared around the globe for their egg, meat, feather and fattened livers. The worldwide population of ducks (*Anas* spp.) is 1.15 billion in 2020 out of which 89 per cent were in Asia. China, Viet Nam, Bangladesh and Indonesia are the largest duck rearing countries in Asia (FAO 2020). Geographical location, subtropical climatic condition, water lodged and low areas of the country are suitable for duck habitat. The advantages of ducks over other poultry species are that they are hardy, have higher disease tolerance and are easy to herd.

Though relatively tolerant to diseases ducks are susceptible to parasitic infection and infestation. Parasites are one of the causes of diseases in ducks and have been reported from different parts of the world including Europe, North America, Asiaand suffer from varieties of parasitic diseases including gastrointestinal helminths, protozoa and external parasites having impact on the productivity and production. The economy of the duck rearing is directly or indirectly affected by parasites in many ways. Heavily parasitized duck results in reduction in food intake, malnutrition, reduction in weight gain, decrease in egg production and lowered fertility. Ducks can act as the final and intermediate hosts for protozoon and helminths parasites.

Geographical factors play an important role in the prevalence of parasitic diseases. The climatic condition suitable for the rearing of ducks also favours the growth and multiplication of various parasites. Managemental practices also play an important role in the transmission of parasitic diseases in ducks. The majority of ducks are reared in the free-range system in the rural areas which predisposes them to parasites.

Helminthic Diseases of Ducks

Helminths are the most prevalent parasites of ducks and have major effects in the productivity. Helminths include the roundworms (nematode), tapeworms (cestode) and flatworms (trematode). These helminths are located in various parts of the gastrointestinal tract including small intestine, large intestine and caecum. The seasonal prevalence of helminths in ducks is almost similar throughout the year but the infectivity rate is the highest in the rainy season as compared to summer and winter months. The rains in the monsoon plays significant role in the propagation of intermediate host such as the snail.

Among the helminths parasites the prevalence of nematode is usually higher in comparison to cestode and trematode. The helminths found in domestic chickens are also usually found in domestic ducks. The presence of infective eggs of the nematode in the environment can indicate the higher prevalence as most nematodes have direct life cycle. Infective eggs can be easily picked up by ducks during feeding and drinking. Ducks reared near running water like streams or rivers also have a higher chance of getting infected. The prevalence of cestode and trematode requires the presence of intermediate host like arthropods and mollusca as they have an indirect life cycle. Area's endemic to the intermediate host can lead to higher infection of ducks by cestodes and trematodes by the ingestion of this infected intermediate host. The transmission and infection of ducks with helminth parasites depend upon the rearing practices as free grazing ducks play important role in the cycle maintenance. Species with direct life cycle are commonly found in intensive system of rearing as they require only optimum temperature and environment for their development. The overall prevalence can be much low in the intensive system of rearing ducks and the low infection can be an indicator of the farm environment, immunity and good managemental practices of the farm.

Heterakiosis

It is a small nematode present in the caecum of birds and characterized by wasting, anemia and diarrhoea.

Etiology

*Heterakis gallinarum*are small to medium sized nematodes that are found in the caeca of birds including ducks. They are non-migrating and one of the most common nematodes found in birds.

Epidemiology

The distribution of *H. gallinarum* is worldwide. It is commonly found in chickens, domesticated turkeys, and many other species of fowl, primarily of poultry. Their eggs are found to live for years in soil making it difficult to eliminate *H. gallinarum* from a domestic flock. Earthworms may ingest the eggs of *H. gallinarum* and contribute to the cause of infections in poultry. Although the eggs are themselves infective, they can develop further into a second infective larval stage. This development occurs around 27 °C and takes 2–4 weeks.

Transmission

H. gallinarum has a direct life cycle not requiring an intermediate host to complete development. *H. gallinarum* is transmitted by direct ingestion of infective eggs from the soil. *Heterakis* eggs are ingested by annelids serving as transport host. Ducks also gets infection by ingestion of the annelids containing second stage of larva. Poultry raised at high density on litter are at risk for accumulating large numbers of the nematode.

Pathogenesis

Pathology of *Heterakis gallinarum* is mild does not significantly affect bird performance but in heavy infection it causes caecal mucosa thickening, appearance of nodules and petechial haemorrhage. *H. gallinarum* is an economically important parasite because of its role in the transmission of the protozoan parasite *Histomonas meleagridis* the cause of Black head disease in poultry resulting in liver disorder and cyanosis of the head of poultry birds.

Clinical findings

The clinical findings are not well marked in *H. gallinarum* infection. Although there may be anaemia, diarrhoea, wasting, emaciation, weakness and decrease in egg production.

Necropsy findings

On examination the adult worms are found in the caeca. Carcass is emaciated, anaemic and lesions are characterized by congestion, petechial hemorrhages of the mucosa thickening of the wall of mucosa, and nodules in the cecal wall of the mucosa.

Diagnosis

Diagnosis of the nematode relies on finding of eggs in the faeces especially the caecal faeces. The eggs should be differentiated with other nematode eggs.

Treatment

Albendazole @ 5 mg/kg b wt once a day for 5 days is effective against most roundworm species in duck and it should be repeated after 10 days. Fenbendazole @ 5-15 mg/kg given orally, once a day for 5 days and it should be repeated after 10 days of intervals. Ivermectin 1% at 10 mg/mL and Levamisole @ 20-

50 mg/kg bodyweight, added to drinking water is effective against nematodes. Pyrantel tartrate @ 15-25 mg/kg b wt of duck is effective against the adult stage of nematodes.

Prevention and control

Ducks can be controlled by keeping birds in hygienic conditions and stopping them wandering around free. Feed and water containers should be cleaned out every day. All the birds should be dewormed atleast before and after breeding every year. Cages and houses should be kept clean with droppings removed every week. The wet muddy areas should be avoided around water containers or anywhere else. Cages and houses should be meticulously cleaned before the entry of new ducklings and birds should not be kept on the same area of ground year after year to avoid the contamination of soil. The different age groups of birds should be kept separately.

Capillariosis

It is caused by *Capillaria* spp. in various species of birds and canimals and characterized by weight loss, enteritis and haemorrhagic diarrhoea.

Etiology

Capillaria annulata, *C. contorta*, *C. bursata* and *C. anatis* are the species of *Capillaria* infecting domestic and wild birds including ducks. The predilection site varies for different species. *Capillaria annulata*, *C. contorta* are found in the crop and oesophagus of birds, *C. bursata* in the small intestine and *C.* anatis in the caecum.

Epidemiology

The prevalance rate of *Capillaria* spp. ranges between 10-15% in ducks.

Transmission

Young birds are more susceptible than adult birds and the adult birds can act as carriers of the disease. Transmission varies between the species as the life cycle varies. The life cycle of *C. annulata* is indirect with the involvement of earthworm as the intermediate host. The eggs passed out along the faeces are ingested by the earthworm and develop into infective larva. Infection occurs by the ingestion of the earthworm harbouring infective larva. *C. contorta*, *C. bursata* and *C. anatis* have direct life cycle with the L1 embryonated egg as the infective stage. Infection occurs by the ingestion of infective eggs along with food and water.

Pathogenesis

Pathogenesis depends upon the species and intensity of infection. Light infection results in mild inflammation, thickening of mucous membranes of the crop and gizzard in infection caused by *Capillaria annulata*, *C. contorta*. Acute infection results in catarrhal inflammation of crop and oesophagus. *C. anatis* infection results in development of infection in the intestines resulting in the anorexia and prostration. *Capillaria* spp. in low numbers may also results in decrease production.

Clinical Findings

Young birds exhibit the most serious clinical signs. Clinical signs include enteritis, weight loss, hemorrhagic and bloody diarrhoea and anaemia.

Necropsy findings

On post mortem examination large numbers of worms can be found in the crop, oesophagus, small and large intestines.

Diagnosis

Diagnosis can be made by examination of faecal sample using faecal floatation techniques demonstrating the un-embryonated bi-operculated eggs of capillaria spp.

Treatment

Ivermectin 1% at 10 mg/mL in water were effective in removing capillaria. Levamisole @ 20-50 mg/kg bodyweight in drinking water is effective against capillaria. Pyrantel tartrate @ 15-25 mg/kg b wt of duck is effective against the adult stage of capillaria.

Prevention and Control

Ducks can be controlled by keeping birds in hygienic conditions and stopping them wandering around free. Feed and water containers should be cleaned out every day. All the birds should be dewormed at least before and after breeding every year. Cages and houses should be kept clean with droppings removed every week. The wet muddy areas should be avoided around water containers or anywhere else. Cages and houses should be meticulously cleaned before the entry of new ducklings and birds should not be kept on the same area of ground year after year to avoid the contamination of soil. The different age groups of birds should be kept separately.

Trichostrongylosis

It is a nematodal parasite present in caecum and small intestine of duck and characterized by diarrhoea mixed with mucus and blood.

Etiology

*Trichostrongylus tenuis*is a nematode located in the caecum and small intestine of chicken and less frequently in ducks. In early stages of infection, it causes diarrhoea from the caeca, later with blood and mucous and ultimately cease to discharge. It causes acute typhlitis but the symptoms are fairly short.

Epidemiology

T. tenuis have low prevalance on domestic ducks. *T. tenuis* is found across Europe, Asia and North America. The eggs and larva can tolerate low temperatures but cannot tolerate high temperature and desiccation.

Transmission

The nematode has a direct life cycle where excreted eggs in the faeces hatch under favourable environmental condition in 36 – 48 hrs. Larvae undergo two moulting to produce the infective L3 larvae in two weeks. Infection is by ingestion of infective L3 larvae which undergoes two moulting in the caecum and small intestine to reach the adult stage.

Pathogenesis

T. tenuis causes inflammation, congestion of blood vessels and extension of mucosa of the caecum. In acute infection there is anaemia and weight loss which can be fatal especially to the young birds.

Clinical findings

Birds affected generally showed depression, diarrhoea, inappetence to anorexia and anaemia.

Diagnosis

Diagnosis can be made by faecal floatation for the demonstration of eggs in the faeces.

Treatment

Albendazole @ 5 mg/kg b wt once a day for 5 days is effective against most roundworm species in duck and it should be repeated after 10 days.

Fenbendazole @ 5-15 mg/kg given orally, once a day for 5 days and it should be repeated after 10 days of intervals.

Prevention and Control

Ducks can be controlled by keeping birds in hygienic conditions and stopping them wandering around free. Feed and water containers should be cleaned out every day. All the birds should be dewormed at least before and after breeding every year. Cages and houses should be kept clean with droppings removed every week. The wet muddy areas should be avoided around water containers or anywhere else. Cages and houses should be meticulously cleaned before the entry of new ducklings and birds should not be kept on the same area of ground year after year to avoid the contamination of soil. The different age groups of birds should be kept separately.

Ascaridiosis

Ascaridiosis in poultry caused by *Ascaridia galli* and characterized by weight loss, diarrhoea and haemorrhagic enteritis.

Etiology

Ascaridiosis is one of the most prevalent helminthiosis in birds including ducks. The ascarid nematode primarily infecting ducks is *Ascaridia galli*. *A. galli* is an ascarid nematode and one of the most commonly reported gastro intestinal parasite of ducks. It is large roundworm located in the small intestine of ducks.

Epidemiology

Ascaridia galli is a common parasite of poultry and has been reported worldwide in chicken, fowl, pigeons, turkey, duck, guinea and goose.

Transmission

A. galli have a direct life cycle and present in the gastrointestinal tract and embryonated eggs in the environment. Infection occurs by the ingestion of infective eggs in the contaminated food and water. Eggs are expellees with the faces where they become infective under favourable environment (temperature and relative humidity). Eggs hatch in the duodenum after 24 hours, the larvae adhere to the intestinal mucosa and ultimately matures in the lumen of intestine. Once it undergoes maturation eggs are passed with the faeces and life cycle continues.

Pathogenesis

A. galli infects birds of all ages, but the most severe damage is found in young birds. Heavy infection is the major cause of weight depression and reduced egg production in poultry husbandry. Severe infections can result in blockage of the small intestine.

Clinical findings

A. galli may cause anorexia, weight loss, haemorrhages in the intestinal mucosa, diarrhoea, obstruction of the intestinal lumen, altered hormone level and eventually death in a wide range of avian species.

Diagnosis

Diagnosis can be made by faecal floatation or direct examination for the demonstration of eggs in the faeces.

Treatment

Albendazole @ 5 mg/kg b wt once a day for 5 days is effective against most roundworm species in duck and it should be repeated after 10 days. Fenbendazole @ 5-15 mg/kg given orally, once a day for 5 days and it should be repeated after 10 days of intervals. Ivermectin 1% at 10 mg/mL in water were effective in removing *A galli*. Levamisole @ 20-50 mg/kg bodyweight, added to drinking water is effective against Ascariasis. Pyrantel tartrate @ 15-25 mg/kg b wt of duck is effective against the adult stage of *A galli*.

Prevention and Control

Ducks can be controlled by keeping birds in hygienic conditions and stopping them wandering around free. Feed and water containers should be cleaned out every day. All the birds should be dewormed at least before and after breeding every year. Cages and houses should be kept clean with droppings removed every week. The wet muddy areas should be avoided around water containers or anywhere else. Cages and houses should be meticulously cleaned before the entry of new ducklings and birds should not be kept on the same area of ground year after year to avoid the contamination of soil. The different age groups of birds should be kept separately.

Echinostomiasis

Echinostomiasis is a zoonotic food- borne intestinal trematode of ducks which is characterized by emaciation and catarrhal enteritis in ducklings.

Etiology

It is caused by *Echinostoma revolutum*, *Echinoparyphium recurvatum*, and *Hypoderaeum conoideum* in ducks. Echinostomes are foodborne and zoonotic intestinal trematodes comprise a group of at least 60 species.

Epidemiology

Echinostomes are zoonotic intestinal trematodes which are found all over the world and endemic in nature. High prevalence of infection with echinostome have been reported in ducks in several south east Asian countries. Echinostoma have 3 host life cycle with snail as first intermediate host. It infects a broad range of host and infection occurs by ingestion of second intermediate hosts, i.e., freshwater snails and fish. The morbidity due to echinostoma depends upon the number of worms present and heavy infection of young duck results in emaciation, catarrhal enteritis and death. The high prevalence of echinostoma depends upon the snail intermediate host present in a particular region and the grazing system used by the farmers. Free grazing ducks acts a reservoir for the echinostomes. These medically important echinostomes infect a broad range of definitive hosts among wild, domestic and peri-domestic animals, e.g., cats, dogs, pigs, rodents, aquatic birds, chickens, and ducks.

Clinical signs

It causes emaciation and catarrhal enteritis and death in young and diseased animals, including ducks.

Diagnosis

The diagnosis is made by identification of large, operculated eggs in stool that are difficult to distinguish from the eggs of *F. hepatica, F. gigantica,* and *F. buski.*

Treatment

Praziquantel @ 25 mg/kg orally as single dose and albendazole @ 400 mg twice daily for 3 days is effective in echinostomes infections.

Prevention and Control

The feeding of raw and improperly cooked freshwater fish and fresh or brackish water snails should be avoided to avoid echinostome metacercarial infections. Control of intermediate host snail using chemical and physical methods.

Echinuriosis

It is caused by small thin nematode *Echinuria uncinata* located in the proventriculus and clinical signs are mostly asymptomatic to emaciation and anaemia in ducks.

Epidemiology

Echinuria is a small, thin nematode that develop in an intermediate host, a water flea or freshwater shrimp. Its outbreaks have reported from many parts of world like United Kingdom, South Amaerica, Canada, Russia, New Zealand in domestic geese and ducks showing the granulomas scattered over the surface of the proventriculus, esophagus, intestine etc. The bird mortality is high in drought areas as high concentration of Daphnia spp. (the intermediate host) in small lakes increases the chance for bird infection. The adult ducks are more resistant to infection as compared the ducklings. Mortalities of wild and domestic birds have been associated to a high intensity of infection by this species and to its high pathogenicity.

Clinical signs

It has been found associated to granulomas, in the esophagus, proventriculus, gizzard, and sometimes, the small intestine. There is thickening of the wall of proventriculus, excessive mucous and nodules in the intestine.

It causes the mucous membrane of the proventriculus to become inflamed and occasionally obstruct the passage of food which impedes the digestion and causes death in severe infestation resulted in death.

Diagnosis

Faecal examination showed the presence of thick shelled elliptical eggs.

Treatment

Albendazole and fenbendazole may be useful.

Management of parasitic diseases in ducks

The recommended management system for is the intensive management system. Proper care and maintenance of the health of ducks against parasitic diseases can be maintained in this system. Good housing system, proper disposal of duck faeces, prevention of contamination of the feeding areas, deworming programme,

We recommend intensive management system for keeping ducks in which adequate care in terms of good housing, routine deworming programme, regular use of anticoccidial drugs and prevention of contamination of environment through hygiene in duck pens and proper disposal of duck faeces and dead ducks could be carried out. These would eliminate or reduce to low level incidence of gastrointestinal parasites and increase duck productivity through increased weight gain, increased feed conversion efficiency and decrease time to reach market weight leading to increase economic gain to farmers

Table 1 : Helminth Parasites of Ducks

Nematode	Cestode	Trematode
Ascaridia galli	*Raillietina* sp.	*Echinostoma* sp.
Heterakis sp.	*Choanotaenia* sp.	*Echinoparyphium*
Capillaria sp.	*Echinolepis carioca*	*E. recurvatum*
Trichuris sp.	*Cladogyniaphoeniconaiadis*	*Echinoparyphiumparaulum*
Strongyloides sp.	*Baerfainiaanoplocephaloides*	*E. revolutum*
Echinuria uncinata	*C. digonopora*	*E. elegans*
Trichostrongylus tenuis	*Sobolevicanthus sp.*	*P. longicirratus*
		Hypodera eumconoideum

References

Adejinmi JO &Oke M (2011). Gastro-intestinal Parasites of Domestic Ducks (Anasplatyrhynchos) in Ibadan Southwestern Nigeria. Asian Journal of Poultry Science5: 46-50.

Begum A, Mukutmoni M & Akter F (2019). Parasite Diversity in Domestic Duck on Anasplatyrhyncosdomestic*us* from *Munshiganj*, Dhaka. Bangladesh Journal of Zoology 47: 121-128.

*Bobrek K, Hild*ebrand J, Urbanowicz J & Gawel A (2019). Molecular Identification and Phylogenetic Analy*sis of Heterakisdispar* Isolated from Geese. Acta Parasitologica 64: 753-760

*Bouz*id M, Hunter PR, Chalmers RM & Tyler KM (2013). Cryptosporidium Pathogenicity and Virulence. Clinical Microbiology Reviews *26: 115-134.*

Callait-Cardinal MP, Chauve C, Reynaud MC, Alogninouwa T, Zenner L. Infectivity of Histomonas meleagridis in ducks. Avian Pathol. 2006 Apr;35(2):109-16. doi: 10.1080/03079450600597626. PMID: 16595302.

Callait-Cardinal MP, Chauve C, Reynaud MC, Alogninouwa T &Zenner L (2006). Infectivi*ty of Histomonasmeleagridis* in ducks. Avian Pathology 35: 109-116.

Cram, E., & Cuvillier, E. (1934). Observations on Trichostrongylustenuis Infestation in Domestic and Game Birds in the United States. Parasitology, 26(3), 340-345. doi:10.1017/S0031182000023659

Cram, E., & Cuvillier, E. (1934). Observations on Trichostrongylus tenuis Infestation in Domestic and Game Birds in the United States. Parasitology, 26(3), 340-345. doi:10.1017/S0031182000023659

Fatoba AJ &Adeleke MA (2018). Diagnosis and control of chicken coccidiosis: a recent update. Journal of Parasitic Diseases 42: 483-493.

Gharagozlou MJ, Mobedi I, Samani RA, TaghizadehF Mowlavi G (2019). Esophageal-Crop Capillariasis and ProventriculusVentriculusHystrichisiasis in a Migratory Duck (*Anascrecca*). Iranian Journal of Parasitology 14: 413-420.

http://www.poultrydvm.com/drugs/albendazole

Hudson, Peter J.; Newborn, David; Dobson, Andrew P. (1992). "Regulation and Stability of a Free-Living Host-Parasite System: Trichostrongylustenuis in Red Grouse. I. Monitoring and Parasite Reduction Experiments". Journal of Animal Ecology. 61(2): 477–486. doi:10.2307/5338. ISSN 0021-8790. Retrieved 18 June 2022.

J.O. Adejinmi and M. Oke, 2011. Gastro-intestinal Parasites of Domestic Ducks (Anasplatyrhynchos) in Ibadan Southwestern Nigeria. Asian Journal of Poultry Science, 5: 46-50.

Kuhn, Ryan C et al. (2002). "Occurrence of Cryptosporidium and Giardia in wild ducks along the Rio Grande River valley in southern New Mexico." Applied and environmental microbiology vol. 68,1: 161-5. doi:10.1128/AEM.68.1.161-165.2002

Larki, Sara, Alireza Alborzi, Rahil Chegini and Rezvan Amiri. (2018). "A Preliminary Survey on Gastrointestinal Parasites of Domestic Ducks in Ahvaz, Southwest Iran." Iranian Journal of Parasitology 13: 137 - 144.

Lima V, Bezerra T, Fonseca de Andrade A, Ramos R, Faustino M, Alves L &Meira-Santos P (2016). Gastrointestinal parasites of exotic birds living in captivity in the state of Sergipe, Northeastern Brazil. Brazilian Journal ofVeterinary Parasitology 26: 96-99.

Lindsay, David S., et al. (1989). "Experimental Infections in Domestic Ducks with Cryptosporidium Baileyi Isolated from Chickens." Avian Diseases, vol. 33, no. 1, pp. 69–73. JSTOR, https://doi.org/10.2307/1591069.

Paul BT, Lawal JR, Ejeh EF, Ndahi JJ, Peter ID, Bello AM & Wakil Y (2015). Survey of Helm*inth Parasites o*f Free Range Muscovy Ducks (Anasplatyrynchos) Slaughtered in Gombe, North Eastern Nigeria. International Journal of Poultry Science 14: 466-470.

Saijuntha W, Duenngai K, Tantrawatpan C. (2013). Zoonotic echinostome infections in free-grazing ducks in Thailand. Korean J Parasitol. 2013 Dec;51(6):663-7. doi: 10.3347/kjp.2013.51.6.663. Epub PMID: 24516271; PMCID: PMC3916455.

Saijuntha W, Duenngai K, Tantrawatpan C. (2013). Zoonotic echinostome infections in free-grazing ducks in Thailand. Korean J Parasitol. 51(6):663-7.

Sharma N, Hunt PW, Hine, BC &Ruhnke I (2019). The impact of Ascaridiagallion performance, health, and immune responses of laying hens: new insights into an old problem. Poultry Science 98: 6517-6526.

Silveira, Eliane& Amato, José & Amato, Suzana.(2006). *Echinuriauncinata* (Rudolphi) (Nematoda, *Acuariidae*) in Nettapeposaca (Vieillot) (Aves, Anatidae) in South America. Revista Brasileira De Zoologia - REV BRAS ZOOL. 23. 10.1590/S0101-81752006000200027.

Soliman, K. (1955). Observations on Some Helminth Parasites from Ducks in Southern England. Journal of Helminthology, 29(1-2), 17-26. doi:10.1017/S0022149X00024172.

Work TM, Meteyer CU, Cole RA. (2004). Mortality in Laysan ducks (Anaslaysanensis) by emaciation complicated by *Echinuriauncinata on* Laysan Island, Hawaii, 1993. J Wildl Dis. 40(1):110-4. doi: 10.7589/0090-3558-40.1.110. PMID: 15137496.

Yazwinski TA & Tucker CA (2008). "Nematod*es* and Acanthocephalans" in Saif YM (ed.) Diseases of Poultry. Blackwell Publishing, Iowa, USA, pp. 1025-1056.

Zajac AM &Conboy GA (2012). "Fecal Exam Procedures" in Zajac AM &Conboy GA (eds.) Veterinary ClinicalParasitology. 8th Edition UK: Wiley-Blackwell, John Wiley & Sons, Inc., pp. 4-15.

12

External Parasites of Ducks

Ducks are prone to several external parasites and are also affected by external parasites found in other poultry birds. Birds are plagued by an remarkable range of ectoparasites, ranging from feather-feeding lice, to feather degrading bacteria and many of these ectoparasites have severe harmful effects on host health. External parasites can make ducks very uncomfortable, transmits several diseases and can be fatal in untreated cases. Among the ectoparasites lice is most commonly found in ducks. Ectoparasites infested birds become restless and the feeding and sleeping is disturbed resulting in decreased growth rate and egg production.

Common ectoparasites present on ducks-

- Fleas
- Lice
- Mites
- Ticks

Fleas

Fleas are small flightless insect which live as external parasites of mammals and avians. Adult fleas are generally brown, extremely small and have flattened sideways or narrow bodies that enables them to move through the fur or feathers of hosts. As it lacks wings, their hind legs are extremely well adapted for jumping. Their mouthparts are adapted for piercing skin and sucking blood of their hosts. These parasites will also bite humans if given the opportunity.

Lice

Ducks are affected by feather lice which is a tiny parasitic insect that invade and live within a duck's feathers. Lice will usually complete their entire life cycle on the duck. In mild infestation lice is usually unnoticed while in severe infestations in young, sick, or injured birds it can cause significant irritation to the bird. In case of intense Irritation There is excessive preening and scratching of their feathers. Ducks affected with lice usually have a dull look to their feathers, which also become ruffled and damaged. In severe loss of feathers, they could die from being too cold. Besides, egg production will decrease, and your bird may lose weight from not eating or resting enough.

Mites

The several species of mites that affects the poultry may also affect the ducks. The common mites that affects the ducks are as

a. **Depluming mite (*Neocnemidocoptes gallinae*):** It is worldwide in distribution and burrows into the epidermis at the base of feather shafts and causing intense irritation and feather pulling and loss in birds in spring and summer. Hyperkeratosis, skin lesions, and digit necrosis can result from the burrowing.

b. **Northern fowl mite (*Ornithonyssus sylviarum*)**: It is an obligate blood-sucking parasites that may live upto 4 weeks off the host and complete life cycle in 5-12 days depending on temperature and relative humidity. This type of mites is generally present in feathers, vent area, which may have thick, crusty skin, severe scabbing, and soiled feathers. In heavy infestations, they can be found on eggs and in moderate infestations it causes decreased egg production and feed conversion efficiency in laying hens.

c. **Red poultry mite (*Dermanyssus gallinae*)**: Red poultry mites populations develop rapidly during the warmer months and more slowly in cold weather. The life cycle may be completed in only 1 week and a house may remain infested for up to 9 months after birds are removed. They are nocturnal feeders that hide during the day under manure, on roosts, and in cracks and crevices of the chicken house, where they deposit eggs. Heavy infestations of red mites decrease reproductive potential in males, egg production in females, weight gain in young birds, and feed conversion efficiency which leads to anemia and death.

d. **Scaly leg mite (*Knemidocoptes mutans*):** It is uncommon in backyard flocks but rare in modern farming, complete entire life cycle in skin and transmitted by contact. Scaly legs mites in older birds causes irritation and exudation in legs which causes legs to become thickened, encrusted and unattractive. Feet and leg scales become raised resulting in lameness, birds stop feeding, occasionally affect comb and wattle and death can result after several months. The entire life cycle is in the skin; transmission is by contact. Infections may remain in latent phase for long periods until stress triggers a mite population increase.

You can find mites on the head and neck of your duck, except for the scaly leg mite, which can cause the legs and feet to be red and swollen. It is easier to see mites on white or light-colored birds, where dark-colored birds can go untreated due to not seeing a visible infestation.

Scaly leg mites can cause lameness and are not typically prevalent in ducks, but it can happen, so knowing what to look for is essential. Other mites can cause skin irritation, loss of feathers, and even death if they are a host for the red poultry mite. If your duck shares a living space with chickens, it could be vulnerable to all these parasites at some time.

Mite infestations occur often in abandoned domestic ducks and wild waterfowl. Mites are a type of ectoparasite (parasite that invades and lives on the outer body of their host), that live within the bird's feathers. Heavy infestations with mites tend to occur in most often in younger, sick, or injured birds. The mites are transmitted to ducks by direct contact with an infected host.

Ticks

The fowl tick or poultry tick (*Argas persicus*) is a small soft-bodied tick which is distributed worldwide in tropical and subtropical countries and is found primarily on domestic fowl such as chickens, ducks, and geese. Ticks of duck range in colour from blue to brown and causes severe problem for ducks if not treated. They are incredibly hardy and live in cracks in walls or trees and can live for several years without feeding on the blood of a bird. Ticks generally bite at night and causes anaemia, weight loss, toxaemia, stop laying eggs and paralysis. The tick bite site is easily recognized by red spots. Fowl ticks are rarely found in commercial cage-layer operations but may be found in cage-free housing, including breeder, pasture, or small-scale flocks.

Prevention and Treatment

Keeping a clean-living area excluding rodents and wild birds from areas where ducks are kept. Quarantine for new birds before introduction in the flocks are useful in prevention of new diseases in flocks. The cages and houses of ducks must be meticulously cleaned. All bedding and dirt must be removed and all parts of the equipment should be thoroughly scrubbed with soap and hot water. The equipment then sprays or paint with a mixture of paraffin and creosote in equal amounts or with nicotine sulphate (40%). Ducks generally clean their feathers daily with soil or sand. The shallow box containing sand and ashes left from a fire are used by birds to keep the feathers clean and free of infections. The light dusting of dusting powder or spray containing, e.g trichlorphon or malathionis useful in minimizing the infestations of ectoparasites specially ticks, fleas and lice in birds. Mite infestations like scaly leg of ducks can be treated by dipping the leg in paraffin (kerosene) and gently brushing it. Prevention of mite introduction in a flock is best because eradication is incredibly difficult in mite infestation in birds. Any acaricidal spray treatments must be applied with sufficient force to penetrate the feathers in the vent area. Dust boxes with sand and acaricidal materials, such as inert dusts like diatomaceous earth or sulfur dust are very effective for bird self-treatment of mites. The 'spot-on' product like ivermectin which kills external parasites is available for pigeons as 1 drop on the skin per 500g of bird weight weekly for 3 weeks may be useful in ducks.

References

Ahmad A, Gupta N, Saxena AK, Gupta DK (2015). Population levels of Phthiraptera on domestic ducks (*Anas platyrhynchos*) (Anseriformes: Anatidae). J Parasit Dis. 39(3):567-71.

Anonymous (2016). CSRTI, Annual report, Central Sericultural Research and Training Institude, Mysore, 17, 19.

Chandra S, Agarwal GP, Singh SPN and Saxena AK (1990). Seasonal changes in a population of Menacanthus eurysternus (Mallophaga, Amblycera) on the common myna Acridotheres tristi. Int J Parasitol.20: 1063-65.

Choi, CY, Takekawa JY, Prosser DJ, Smith, L.M., Ely, C.R., Fox, AD, Kao, L, Wang, X., Batbayar, N., Natsagdorj, T and Xiao, X (2016). Chewing Lice of Swan Geese (Anser cygnoides). New Host-Parasite Associations. The Korean Journal of Parasitology. 54(5):685-91.

Clayton DH and Drown DM (2001). Critical evaluation of five methods for quantifying chewing lice (Insecta: phthiraptera). J Parasitol. 87: 1291-300.

Clayton DH and Tompkins DM (1994). Ectoparasite virulence is linked to mode of transmission. Proc R Soc Lond B Biol., 256: 211- 17.

Eveleigh ES and Threlfall W (1976). Population dynamics of lice (*Mallophaga*) on auks (Alcidae) from newfoundland. Can J Zool., 54: 1694-711.

Flinchum, Gwen (2014). Management of Waterfowl Clinical Avian Medicine. 69 .832-848.

Harbison CW, Bush SE, Malenke JR and Clayton DH (2008). Comparative transmission dynamics of competing parasite species. *Ecology*, 89: 3186-94.

Lee PLM and Clayton DH (1995). P opulation biology of swift (*Apus Apus*) ectoparasites in relation to host reproductive success. Ecol Entomol., 20: 43-50.

McGroarty DL and Dobson RC (1974). Ectoparasite populations on house sparrows in northwestern indiana, Am Midl Nat. 91: 479-86.

Susan E. Aiello and Michael A. Moses (2019). The Merck Veterinary Manual. Merck, 11th Edn, John Wiley & Sons, USA.

13

Wild Ducks and Their Diseases

India is a "Winter / Summer Home" for most of the Siberian birds such as Siberian Cranes, Greater Flamingo and Demoiselle Crane, also numerous species of birds from other regions of the world. These beautiful birds migrate to India every year during the winter and summer season for food, breeding and nesting. The migratory birds mainly arriving from Siberia and South East Asia move to the different wetland spots of the national parks/ wildlife sanctuaries etc. in India and are also seen in parts of the lakes and settling down in shallow or fresh water ponds. In the Indian subcontinent, more than 220 types of migratory birds can be found every year, most of them choose the Indian subcontinent as their wintering ground, though some of them are monsoon and summer visitors. They come here from different corners of the world – some of them come from Arctic tundra region; some of them come from Europe, Northern Asia, and even from Iceland. But not all migratory birds do long-distance migrations, some bird species are short-distance migrant in nature; they travel only some hundreds of miles in search of better food resources. In the Indian subcontinent some short-distance migrants of Himalaya change their altitude only, in response to the weather condition – this is called altitudinal migration.

Important migratory ducks encountered in wet lands of India-

Lot of wetlands in Gujarat and Bharatpur are the first stop for most of the migratory birds. "Saurashtra gets the common and demoiselle cranes. Bharatpur in Rajasthan and Khijadiya in Gujarat. Jamnagar has wetlands and coastal birds. Migratory ducks fly to Bharatpur and also to Vedanthangal in Tamil Nadu state. Important migratory species of ducks related to India are furnished below:

- Ruddy shelducks (Syn: Brahminy Ducks in India)
- Garganey dabbling ducks
- Falcated ducks (these are the dabbling ducks)
- Gadwall ducks
- Comb Ducks

Commonly found ducks in the wildlife areas (esp.the wet lands) of India are-

Pink headed ducks, Lesser Whistling Duck, Northern Shoveler, Indian Spot Billed duck, Norther Pintail, Eurasian teal, Common Pochard, Garganey Duck, Tufted Duck, Knob billed duck, Falacted Duck, Mallard Duck.

The goose birds found in India include Bar headed goose, Greylag goose, Cotton pygmy goose, white fronted goose, Red breasted goose, bean goose and swans include Mute swan, Tundra swan and Whooper swan.

In this context, it appears worthy to understand about the important migratory species of India also and they comprise the Taiga Flycatchers, Northern Pintail, Indian Pittas, Blue-fronted Redstart, Wagtails, Bluethroat, Curlew Sandpiper, Siberian Rubythroats, Cotton Pygmy Goose, Greylag goose, Siberian Cranes, Demoiselle Crane, Greater Flamingo, Great White Pelican, Amur Falcon, Bar-headed Goose, Black-winged Stilt, Blue-tailed Bee-eater, Rosy Starling etc.

The winter visitors to India comprise the Black-tailed Godwit, Ruddy Shelduck, Osprey, Pallid Harrier, Eurasian Sparrow Hawk, Common Starling, White Wagtail etc. The summer visitors to India comprise the Jacobin Cuckoo (or) pied crested cuckoo (it is partially migratory bird in India), Comb Duck, Lesser whitethroat, Kingfisher, Blue Tailed Bee Eater, Eurasian Golden Oriole, Black Crowned Night Heron etc. Higher temperature and high-water levels due to good monsoon might have led to an increase in intra-species and inter-species competition for resources.

The weaker individuals, exhausted from the long journey, perhaps were unable to compete, and may have succumbed to stress emanating from the shortage of food, susceptibility to disease/pollutants/toxins and other habitat-related factors in the wintering grounds. In such an eventuality, it is expected that with fall of temperature and lowering of water levels, the incidence of such mortality will go down.

The clinical signs exhibited by affected birds might often include dullness, depression, anorexia, flaccid paralysis in legs and wings, and neck touching the ground. The birds might frequently be unable to walk, swim (or) take flight. Deficit in locomotion (in land and in water-stagnated wet-lands) including swimming and flight are evident, in general; sometimes, the flying capacity may be reduced i.e.there is a compromise in the flying performance of the ducks in sky. Additionally, the disease affected birds may reveal dropped neck, and severe dyspnoea.

The best way to protect waterfowl from catastrophic disease outbreaks is to conserve an abundance of high-quality habitat in areas visited by large numbers of birds. By protecting, restoring, and enhancing wetlands in these areas, one can attempt to prevent the unhealthy concentrations of waterfowls including the wild ducks from gathering on limited habitats. This reduces the birds' susceptibility to infections as well as the potential for the disease to spread throughout the larger waterfowl population.

Diseases of ducks affecting birds around the world can be conveniently divided based on the causal agent. Nevertheless, the basic rules of biosecurity and disease control apply to the prevention of most diseases, whatever the causal organism.

Avian Influenza (AI) in Wild Ducks (Bird Flu)

Birds are the natural hosts for Avian Influenza viruses. Bird flu (or) Avian Influenza, is a viral infection spread from bird to bird. Currently, a particularly deadly strain of bird flu -- H5N1 -- continues to spread among poultry in Egypt and in certain parts of Asia. Technically, H5N1 is a highly pathogenic avian influenza (HPAI) virus. It's deadly to most birds.

Etiology

Avian influenza (bird flu) refers to disease caused by infection with avian (bird) influenza (flu) Type A viruses. The Avian Influenza virus belongs to the family: Orthomyxoviridae and is generally divided into followings:

- Influenza A (occurring in multiple species)
- Influenza B (occurring in homosapiens)
- Influenza C (homosapiens and swines)

Specific bird flu viruses are classified and differentiated from one another by their genetic properties.

Avian influenza A viruses are classified into following two categories:

1. Highly pathogenic avian influenza (HPAI) A viruses.
2. Low pathogenicity avian influenza (LPAI) A viruses.

Many of the recently reported H5N1 bird flu viruses causing infections in wild birds and poultry in the United States belong to clade 2.3.4.4b.

Note

- Most swine influenza viruses do not cause disease in humans, but some countries have reported cases of human infection from certain swine influenza viruses. Close proximity to infected pigs or visiting locations where pigs are exhibited has been reported for most human cases, but some limited human-to-human transmission has occurred.
- Just like birds and pigs, other animals such as horses and dogs, can be infected with their own influenza viruses (canine influenza viruses, equine influenza viruses, etc.).

Epidemiology

Only viruses of the Influenza virus A genus have been isolated from birds and termed avian influenza [AI] viruses, but viruses with all 16 haemagglutinin [H1-H16] and all 9 neuraminidase [N1-N9] influenza A subtypes in the majority of possible combinations have been isolated from avian species. Since the 1990s AI infections due to two subtypes have been widespread in poultry across a large area of the World. LPAI H9N2 appears to have spread across the whole of Asia in that time and has become endemic in poultry in many of the affected countries. After an outbreak of A (H5N1) virus in 1997 in poultry in Hong Kong SAR, China, since 2003, these avian and other influenza viruses have spread from Asia to Europe and Africa. In 2013, human infections with the influenza A(H7N9) virus were reported in China.

However, these outbreaks have tended to have been overshadowed by the H5N1 HPAI virus, initially isolated in China that has now spread in poultry and/or wild birds throughout Asia and into Europe and Africa, resulting in the death or culling of hundreds of millions of poultry and posing a significant zoonosis threat. Airborne transmission may occur if birds are in close proximity and with appropriate air movement.

Swine appear to be important in the epidemiology of infection of turkeys with swine influenza virus when they are in close proximity. Other mammals do not appear to be involved in the epidemiology of HPAI. The infection of humans with an H5 avian influenza virus in Hong Kong in 1997 has resulted in a reconsideration of the role of the avian species in the epidemiology of human influenza.

Wild birds have been implicated in the expansion of highly pathogenic avian influenza virus (H5N1) outbreaks across Asia, the Middle East, Europe, and Africa (in addition to traditional transmission by infected poultry, contaminated equipment, and people). Such a role would require wild birds to excrete virus in the absence of debilitating disease. By experimentally infecting wild ducks, it was found that tufted ducks, Eurasian pochards, and mallards excreted significantly more virus than common teals, Eurasian wigeons, and gadwalls; yet only tufted ducks and, to a lesser degree, pochards became ill or died. These findings suggest that some wild duck species, particularly mallards, can potentially be long-distance vectors of highly pathogenic avian influenza virus (H5N1) and that others, particularly tufted ducks, are more likely to act as sentinels.

Incidence

The bird flu viruses have been identified in more than 100 different species of wild birds, around the world and outbreaks are more common with domestic poultry. However, the wild aquatic avian species like the gulls, terns and shorebirds, in addition to the wild waterfowl such as ducks, geese and swans are considered as the natural reservoirs ie. natural hosts for the bird flu viruses (Avian influenza viruses). Some bird flu viruses have infected other mammalian species, and rarely, sporadic human infections with some bird flu viruses had been documented.

The largest increase in HPAI A(H5N1) virus outbreaks in poultry and wild birds occurred during 2004-2006.

It is to be noted that mutations are often noticed in domestic poultry and no elaborative research has been carried out in many water fowl species, including the wild ducks, in this regard.

Transmission

Bird flu generally spreads through various kinds like the secretions from nasal passages in addition to the eyes, saliva and droppings in case of water fowls and however, it does not necessarily lead to the massive die-offs in case of wild ducks and geese. In this context, the wild ducks and geese are also amenable for the occurrence of bird flu, like the case with other water fowls. However, the bird flu is common among the domestic chicken and turkeys, in general and it seems worthwhile to mention that in case of poultry, genetic mutations of these viruses do occur; in this context, some low-pathogenic viruses can undergo mutation into highly pathogenic avian influenza viruses.

These viruses occur naturally among wild aquatic birds worldwide and can infect domestic poultry and other bird and animal species. Wild aquatic birds include waterbirds (waterfowl) such as ducks, geese, swans, gulls, and terns, and shorebirds, such as storks, plovers, and sandpipers. Wild aquatic birds, especially dabbling ducks, are generally highly found to be the reservoirs (hosts) for these avian influenza A viruses. Wild aquatic birds can be infected with avian influenza A viruses in their intestines and respiratory tract, but some species, such as ducks, may not get sick. However, avian influenza A viruses are very contagious among birds, and some of these viruses can sicken and even kill certain domesticated bird species, including chickens, ducks and turkeys.

In this context, it becomes noteworthy to mention that the insects and rodents may mechanically carry these viral antigens from the wild ducks of infected group to the ducks of non-infected group. Vertical type of transmission shall be suspected always in case of influenza viral outbreaks when it occurs. Influenza virus has also been recovered from the water samples and organic materials that are collected from or at the site of water bodies.

Co-mingling of different birds in the water bodies esp. during the migratory seasons is again to be considered as one of the concrete factors related to the transmission of this viral disease, among the wild ducks. According to the U.S. Centers for Disease Control and Prevention, the risk to public health from the outbreak of Avian influenza is low.

The dynamics of the spread of avian influenza viruses are very complex and the HPAI is a trans-boundary disease, which indicates that it is highly contagious and spreads rapidly across national borders. Detection of these HPAI viruses in wild birds has been revealed currently and reports may coincide with migratory seasons of the water fowls in the concerned geographical region.

Link of Migratory ducks to avian influenza virus infections in poultry, turkey and game birds

It involves serious kinds of research to have a concrete link between the period of occurrence of avian influenza virus infections among the domestic birds (domestic poultry, turkeys and game birds) and the period of migratory activity i.e. migratory season related to the wild waterfowls like wild ducks, wild geese etc.

Documentations on occurrence of HPAI in wild birds of Asia, Europe and Africa are available and it is to be noted that many migratory bird species travel thousands of miles between continents, posing a continuing risk of avian influenza virus transmission.

The comb ducks are found in the wetlands of Africa, Madagascar and India. Falcated ducks are dabbling ducks (A dabbling duck is a type of shallow water duck that feeds primarily along the surface of the water or by tipping headfirst into the water to graze on aquatic plants, vegetation, larvae, and insects and dabbling ducks are the freshwater ducks which typically feed in shallow water by dabbling and upending, such as the mallard, teal, and pintail; Northern Pintail is a migratory duck wintering in India. Pintail prefers the habitats of shallow and freshwater ponds, lakes and backwaters of dams) which concretely belong to the migratory groups of birds in India. These ducks migrate through the Atlantic Ocean and spend winter in Uttar Pradesh, Bihar and Assam.

Gadwalls are very common duck species in northern America and northern Europe. They are long-distance migrants and can be found in wetlands of the Indian subcontinent during winters.

Ruddy shelducks which are also called as Brahminy Ducks in India are also migratory in nature Indian subcontinent (During winter seasons, they migrate to the Indian subcontinent from central Asia and Europe).

Pathogenesis

Only some avian influenza A (H5) and avian influenza A (H7) viruses have been grouped as HPAI A viruses, whereas most avian influenza A (H5) and avian influenza A (H7) viruses which are existing by circulation among birds are LPAI A viruses.

Avian influenza virus belongs to the family of highly contagious viruses that are not harmful to wild birds that transmit it, but are deadly to domesticated birds (poultry, turkey and game birds), in general.

Followings are the significant pathogenic changes noticed in the affected birds

Lesions reflect the patho-physiological damage to the respiratory, digestive and reproductive systems. Visceral organs esp. the brain, heart and pancreas (pancreatic congestion and ulcerations) are highly affected.

Clinical findings

The bird flu viruses can infect the respiratory and gastrointestinal tract of birds. Being the natural reservoirs in the wild, the water fowls like wild ducks and geese do not typically get sick, when they are infected with it. However, it is opposite in case of poultry including turkeys in which cases, during their direct (or) indirect contact with faeces of infected wild birds (often the aquatic avian species), they get infected, starting to reveal clinical symptoms like the depression, coughing and sneezing and sudden death.

In many occasions, the wild birds act just as carriers and symptoms may not be much apparent which perhaps mean that the aquatic avian species esp. water fowls act as symptomless carriers. The disease may run from mild form to severely fatal form.

Inherent pathogenicity of the viral antigen, species and age of the water fowls become the determining factors for the occurrence of this viral infection, in addition to the environmental factors.

However, followings have been quoted as the important clinical symptoms of avian flu in general:

- Ruffled feather
- Droopiness
- Incoordination
- Loss of ability to walk and to stand.
- Complete paralysis
- Swelling around the eyes

- Blood-tinged discharge from the nostrils
- Twisting of the head and neck,
- Particularly, affected ducks may reveal depression, head shaking, torticollis, in-coordination, paralysis and diarrhoea

In general, most of the avian Influenza A viruses are low pathogenic and the occurrence of such low pathogenic avian influenza A viruses cause few signs of diseases in the associated aquatic wild bird species, like ruffled feathers and reduction in laying of eggs, as extrapolated from poultry sector.

In wild ducks, followings are noticed as clinical symptoms specifically

- Labored breathing
- Increased recumbency
- Neurologic signs (torticollis, circling, loss of balance, and head tremors).

Necropsy findings

- Ecchymosis of shank and feet
- Oedema of the head and discoloration of the skin
- Inflammation of the sinuses, trachea and air sacs.
- Haemorrhages in internal organs esp. in ovaries and oviducts
- Ulcerations in the gastro-intestinal tract
- Enlargement of the spleen

Diagnosis

The disease is diagnosed by clinical symptoms and by usage of the molecular diagnostics such as polymerase chain reaction (PCR) tests, Real time-PCR, virus isolation and controlled laboratory challenge of experimental birds of the same group.

Serological diagnosis shall be made, based on AGID, HI tests and ELISA tests. The BSL-4 Laboratory of ICAR i.e. the High Security Animal Disease Laboratory of HPAI at Bhopal is the *OIE*-recognized reference-laboratory towards making a proper diagnosis of the avian influenza virus in India and hence, the clinical samples and the samples obtained from the post-mortem of the wild ducks if any need to be sent to this laboratory for arriving at a diagnosis of avian influenza viral infection in them.

Differential diagnosis: The disease is to be differentiated with diseases affecting nervous system and bacterial infections, in general.

Treatment: The disease is not much amenable for treatment, in general.

Prevention and Control

- Capture the affected birds with clinical symptoms and isolate them for effecting the control of disease. It is to be noted that the recovered birds too can shed the viral antigens in an intermittent manner.
- Disposal of carcass instantly in a hygienic manner.
- Wear gloves whenever post-mortem is carried out in case of wild ducks as well as wild geese and wear spectacles also to avoid accidental spilling of secretions or discharges from the wild ducks/geese.
- Prevent the contacts between wild aquatic ducks or any aquatic wild birds and domestic poultry because of the reason that the water fowls are the natural reservoirs of this viral infection.
- Adapt suitable bio-security measures.

Duck Virus Hepatitis

Duck viral hepatitis is an acute and per-acute, highly contagious, viral disease of young ducklings characterized by a short incubation period, sudden onset, high mortality and characteristic liver lesions.

Etiology

Duck hepatitis A virus (DHAV) is one of the pathogens that cause fatal duck viral hepatitis (DVH) in ducklings, which is an acute and contagious disease with a high mortality rate. This disease is caused by the duck hepatitis virus, a highly infectious disease and this is a virus of genus Enterovirus and belongs to the family of Picornaviridae. Outbreaks are frequent in duck flocks with access to bodies of water cohabited with free-living waterfowl.

Duck hepatitis A virus genotype C (DHAV-C), recognized recently, is one of the pathogens causing fatal duck viral hepatitis in ducklings, especially in Asia. Duck viral hepatitis (DVH) is an acute, highly contagious, viral disease typically affecting ducklings of less than six weeks of age. DVH is characterized by a short incubation period, sudden onset, high mortality, and characteristic liver lesions. The viruses that cause DVH in ducklings should not be confused with duck hepatitis B virus, a hepadnavirus infection of older ducks.

The originally described, most widespread, and most virulent subtype of duck viral hepatitis, traditionally referred to as DVH Type I, has been renamed duck hepatitis A virus type 1 (DHAV-1) and is now classified in the genus *Avihepatovirus* in the Picornaviridae family. DHAV is readily propagated in chicken and duck embryos, and they do not produce hemagglutinins.

Viruses that differ from DHAV have been recognized as causes of DVH in ducklings. DVH Type II, now classified as duck astrovirus type 1 (DAstV-1), is difficult to propagate under laboratory conditions; DVH Type III is also now classified as an astrovirus (DAstV-2) and can be propagated in duck (but not chicken) embryos.

Epidemiology

The virus causing duck viral enteritis is mainly transmitted by direct contact from infected to susceptible ducks or by indirect contact with a contaminated environment. Wild birds may play an important role in the spread of the virus, because they can transmit the virus mechanically. Specific antibodies were found in wild ducks living in the immediate vicinity of ducks for breeding. Two antigenically distinct genotypes have been identified in Taiwan (DHAV-2) and identified in China and South Korea (DHAV-3).

Although adults may become infected, clinical signs have not been seen in ducks >7 weeks old, even though the ducklings get affected at the age of 1-4 weeks of age. Duck viral hepatitis (DHV) is on the list of diseases notified to the World Organization for Animal Health (OIE). The disease has been described for the first time in ducks in the United States in the 1950s. Currently, it is noted in many countries around the world. In Poland, duck viral hepatitis was described for the first time in the 1960s and 1970s.

Wild birds could be mechanical carriers. A virus closely related to duck hepatitis B virus (DHBV) was isolated from serum and liver samples of wild migratory ducks (mallards) caught in two separate wildlife reserve parks in France. The wild mallard strain DHBV was experimentally transmitted to mallard and Pekin ducklings and induced a chronic viraemia in both varieties of infected birds. This strain might be the common ancestor of all DHBV strains isolated from domestic ducks world-wide. The discovery of a DHBV-related virus in the natural wild population might be an important clue in the study of the different roles of environmental, host and viral factors in the pathogenesis of DHBV infection, and their possible oncogenic action in ducks.

There is often more than 90% mortality in the affected ducklings. At the same time, mortality of about 10% may also be noticed in some instances. Hence, variations in the rate of mortality shall be anticipated in any incidences of encountering the duck virus hepatitis.

Transmission

The infection occurs mainly by ingestion. Less important is infection through the respiratory system. Water seems to be a natural route of viral transmission.

Outbreaks are frequent in duck flocks with access to bodies of water cohabited with free-living waterfowl. Parenteral, intranasal, or oral administration of infected tissues can establish experimental infection. A carrier condition is suspected in wild birds. And the recovered birds become latently infected carriers and may shed the virus periodically.

Pathogenesis

Incubation period of this disease is more than 24 hours. The pathogenicity of duck viral hepatitis virus becomes increasingly severe with length of time after the infection. Apoptotic cells get ubiquitously distributed, especially among lymphocytes, macrophages and monocytes in immune organs such as the bursa of Fabricius, thymus and spleen, and in liver, kidney and cerebral cells.

One might observe the necrosis in most of the organs and the changes might be characterized by cell swelling and collapsed plasma membrane. The findings generally indicate that the causal organism of this duck virus hepatitis in ducks (often the cause is DHAV-C virus) is pantropic, causing apoptosis and necrosis of different organs. The apoptosis and necrosis caused by the DHAV-C field strain generally associate with the pathogenesis DHAV-C-induced lesions.

Clinical findings

The incubation period for DHAV-1 is 18–48 hours. Affected ducklings become lethargic, lose balance, paddle spasmodically, and die within minutes, typically with opisthotonos. Mortality may be as high as 95% in fully susceptible ducklings. Practically all deaths occur within 1 week after onset of signs. One characteristic sign of affected ducklings is that they fall on their sides, paddle their legs and involved in arching of back of neck, often in opisthotonus. However, depression and greenish diarrhoea may be noticed.

Necropsy findings

The lesions caused by all three types of DVH are similar. The carcass of birds may often reveal enlarged and mottled liver and liver may be covered with hemorrhagic foci of up to 1 cm in diameter. Many times, the hepatic structures may reveal numerous and cellular infiltrations, in addition to the necrotic changes. The spleen may be enlarged and mottled. Kidneys may be swollen, and renal blood vessels congested.

Diagnosis

The disease shall be confirmed by the virus neutralization and PCR. This viral antigen shall be detected in the liver and Fluorescent Antibody Test (FAT) shall be of use in the effective diagnosis of this disease. Viral isolation shall be carried out from hepatic tissues, faeces and whole blood by inoculating into the embryonated eggs in which case, about 60% of the infected embryos die within five days, revealing stunted growth, oedema and greenish discoloration of the embryo fluid.

DHAV-1 may be isolated in duck embryos and duck-embryo liver cell cultures, or less easily in chicken embryos. The virus can also be identified by virus neutralization with specific antisera or by inoculation into both susceptible and immune day-old ducklings. DAstV-1 and DAstV-2 are not neutralized by classic DHAV-1 antiserum. DHAV, DAstV-1, and DAstV-2 can be identified by reverse transcriptase (RT) PCR. Several multiplex RT-PCR tests have been developed for differentiation of the DHAV genotypes.

Differential diagnosis

The disease is to be differentiated from bacterial affections associated with liver by appropriate culture and PCR

Treatment

The disease is difficult to carry out in free ranging regions.

Prevention and Control

- Periodic capture and checking of young ducks / ducklings if available in the concerned water bodies of free ranging wildlife regions.
- Due disposal of dead birds in water bodies
- Barriers need to be placed around water bodies depending on practical possibilities in the event of severe outbreaks among wild fowls including the ducks.

Duck Plague (Syn: Duck Virus Enteritis)

The duck virus enteritis disease (DVE) causes acute type of disease with high mortality rates in the flocks of ducks, geese and swans.

Etiology

The disease is a contagious disease and if often fatal and is caused by the herpes virus (Anatid Herpes Virus). Duck viral enteritis is a **worldwide disease caused by Anatid alpha herpesvirus-1 (AnHV-1)** of the family Herpesviridae that causes acute disease with high mortality rates in flocks of ducks, geese, and swans.

Antigenically, many types are homogenous antigenically, but often they may differ in terms of virulence. High and persistent mortality occur with this viral disease in wild duck like water fowls.

Epidemiology

It is worldwide in distribution. It is spread both vertically and horizontally-through contaminated water and direct contact. Migratory waterfowl are a major factor in the spread of this disease as they are often asymptomatic carriers of disease. The incubation period is three to seven days. This disease is not a zoonotic disease. This disease is noticed during the spring seasons across the world. The USA, Netherlands and UK have incidences like this mostly from March to June.

The DVE disease was first reported in West Bengal earlier and high incidences (40.0%) of DVE have been reported since then. In November 1976, this disease was reported in Tamil Nadu with high mortality (up to 100%) among Indian Runner ducks and later in Tirunelveli district of Tamil Nadu. At the same time, an outbreak of DVE was reported at Kerala state in 1976, wherein disease spread was noticed in all parts of Kerala within a short span of 3-4 months.

The first outbreak of DVE, affecting both ducklings and adult ducks of both sexes was reported in Assam in 1978 with high morbidity (100% in ducklings and between 88-90% in adult birds) and mortality (49% in adult birds). This disease is most often observed in ducks that are older in the age group. Rarely, it is also noticed among the ducklings and the ducks as young as one week old can be infected

Transmission

The disease spreads by direct and indirect contacts, particularly through the water due to the movement of the aquatic birds in ponds, lakes and other water bodies esp. in the stagnated water bodies. Solid natural immunity develops in recovered birds.

Pathogenesis

Duck plague attacks the vascular system, causing haemorrhages and death mostly occurs within fourteen days subsequent to the exposure. The transmission of duck plague occurs mainly through the bird-to-bird contact, among the group of ducks in that wildlife region.

Clinical findings

Wild ducks may die in good condition at the water bodies and mortality rate may even go to 90 per cent.

However, following clinical symptoms may be noticed in the affected ones-

- Reduction or failure of swimming capacity
- Nervous symptoms occur and often paralysis of legs and wings is encountered.
- Lachrymation
- Depression
- Greenish diarrhoea

Necropsy findings

Hepatic structures are generally affected and the lesions may be encountered in the hepatic tissues with enlargement in addition to the specific punctate type of lesions or ecchymotic haemorrhagic lesions. Reddish to brownish discolorations (copper colored liver is noticed frequently in the affected birds) are noticed on the surface of liver which often becomes pale in appearance and there may be an enlargement of spleen and often, kidneys may get swollen with presence of congestions at the renal blood vessels.

Ulcers are present in the gastro-intestinal tract and sometimes; diphtheritic deposits are noticed in the mucous membrane of oesophagus. Most of the time, despite the differences in genotypes, the lesions are of similar in nature among the affected ducks.

Blood in body cavities and petechiae in many organs are witnessed in the affected birds.

Diagnosis

The disease is by clinical symptoms and isolation of the viral antigen in CCL -141 cell line and duck embryo fibroblasts. The confirmatory diagnosis includes inoculation of DPV into ducklings, propagation into chorio-allantoic membrane (CAM) of embryonated duck eggs and isolation of the virus on cell cultures / cell lines derived from ducklings followed by identification by DPV-specific gene segment by PCR targeting various genes such as UL30 and US4 (gD) gene, restriction fragment length polymorphism (RFLP) and nucleotide sequencing.

The demonstration of virus shall be supported by carrying out the fluorescent antibody tests and appropriate ELISA tests.

Differential diagnosis

The disease is to be differentiated from diarrhoea due to any other organism like *Salmonella* (or) *E'coli* infections and appropriate culture and chemical tests in addition to PCR shall help in differential diagnosis

Treatment

The treatment disease is not possible successfully. However, high valued ducks shall be captured by appropriate procedures and broad-spectrum antibiotics like fluoroquinolone compound shall be administered. The drug - Resveratrol has shown to have some antiviral activity against this virus.

Prevention and Control

- Attempts to minimize or avoid the usage of the contaminated water source in free ranging regions shall be made.
- The hygienic disposal of carcasses is to be meticulously carried out in time.

Western Equine Encephalitis

Western Equine encephalitis is one of many mosquito-transmitted viral infections that may progress to acute inflammation of the brain parenchyma and meninges. It is caused by an Alphavirus, which is spread primarily by the bite of the *Culex* and *Aedes* species of mosquito, or possibly by small, wild mammals. Birds are a reservoir but not a primary vector for the virus. It has zoonotic significance and in the human beings, adults are more commonly targeted by the vector but have lower infectivity rates. However, when they are infected, older adults are more likely to develop more severe, neuroinvasive disease (or) to die; infants and very young children are also more likely to develop the neurologic manifestations of the disease and seizures. They are more likely than adults to develop permanent disability after infection. The virus is transmitted into the subcutaneous tissue of the host via the bite of an infected mosquito. The virus then begins replication and synthesis of RNA and protein, usually in the local lymph nodes. Viremia ensues, and if the viral load is high enough, the virus may translocate into the central nervous system across the blood-brain barrier resulting in cerebral and meningeal inflammation and necrosis. Most cases are associated with epidemics in birds or horses. Preventive measures against the bite of mosquitoes are the specific measure useful for the prevention of this viral infection.

Eastern Equine Encephalitis Virus (EEE)

Eastern Equine Encephalitis virus (EEE) is an arbovirus which is a mosquito-borne virus. It circulates between bird reservoir hosts and mosquitoes. Most infected animals and people have inapparent infections, but EEE can cause mortality in some species of birds such as pigeons, pheasants, emus and other species of wild birds. The majority of wild birds infected with the virus will exhibit no clinical signs. Mammals are incidental hosts and humans and horses are the most common mammals to develop clinical disease. EEE has also caused illness in pigs, rodents, and white-tailed deer. Transmission occurs from the bite of an infected mosquito. Mosquitos become infected with EEE when they take a blood meal from a bird that is carrying the virus. Mosquitos then transmit the virus to other birds during subsequent blood meals, continuing the cycle. EEE is not transmitted by direct contact. The virus can be diagnosed by laboratory testing of blood, tissues, or cerebrospinal fluid. There is no cure for EEE and supportive care is the only treatment for neuro-invasive (severe) EEE.

Venezuelan Equine Encephalitis (VEE)

This is also caused like the earlier encephalitis related viral infections, by the members of the family Togaviridae and belong to the genus Alpha virus. Venezuelan equine encephalitis (VEE) is a viral, vector-borne disease in horses and humans in Central America, South America, Mexico and occasionally the southern United States that causes inflammation of the brain. The VEE virus is related to the viruses that cause Eastern and Western equine encephalitis. More than 100 species of birds have been either virologically (or) serologically associated with transmission of epidemic VEE virus. Shore birds in general and herons in particular appear to be capable of serving as amplifier hosts. Eastern and Western equine encephalitis are typically spread from birds to horses by mosquito vectors, but are not transmitted between horses by mosquitoes. Conversely, if a mosquito bites a horse infected with VEE, there is enough virus in the blood that it can be transmitted to another horse that the mosquito bites. Rodents are the natural hosts for the VEE virus, but birds may be involved in some cases. Since aerosolized VEE can cause fatal encephalitis in humans, it is considered a possible bio-warfare agent.

Japanese Encephalitis

Japanese encephalitis is caused by a virus and it is transmitted by the bite of **Culex mosquitoes.** The transmission of the disease is maintained by egrets and other aquatic birds most of which are migratory and by pigs which are the amplifier hosts. There is no human-to-human transmission.

Japanese encephalitis virus (JEV) is a flavivirus related to dengue, yellow fever and West Nile viruses, affecting man and the JEV is transmitted to humans through bites from infected mosquitoes of the *Culex* species (mainly *Culex tritaeniorhynchus*). Humans, once infected, do not develop sufficient viraemia to infect feeding mosquitoes.

Linkage between water birds and Japanese encephalitis

The virus exists in a transmission cycle between mosquitoes, pigs and/or water birds (enzootic cycle). The disease is predominantly found in rural and peri-urban settings, where humans live in closer proximity to these vertebrate hosts. In most temperate areas of Asia, JEV is transmitted mainly during the warm season, when large epidemics can occur. In the tropics and subtropics, transmission can occur year-round but often intensifies during the rainy season and pre-harvest period in rice-cultivating regions. Human beings are affected by epidemics of Japanese encephalitis virus is Southeast Asia, India, Korea, China, and Indonesia and mainly affects children, with a mortality of about 30%. In peri-domestic settings, pigs and aquatic wading birds are reported to be the natural as amplifying / reservoir hosts of Japanese encephalitis virus-transmission and aquatic birds as maintenance hosts of the virus.

Japanese encephalitis virus (JEV) is the most common cause of acute encephalitis syndrome (AES) in many countries including India. The first case of Japanese encephalitis viral disease (JE) was documented in 1871 in Japan. This disease often occurs in outbreaks. Japanese encephalitis (JE) was first reported in India among human beings in 1955 when clinical cases were reported from the cities of Vellore and Pondicherry in southern India. Since then, the disease has spread to West Bengal, Uttar Pradesh, Assam, Manipur, Bihar, Andhra Pradesh, Pondicherry, Karnataka, Goa, Kerala and Maharashtra, and in recent years its prevalence has been most notable in Uttar Pradesh and its neighbouring state of Bihar which are located in north India

The annual incidence of clinical disease varies both across and within endemic countries, ranging from <1 to >10 per 100 000 population or higher during outbreaks. A literature review estimates nearly 68 000 clinical cases of JE globally each year, with approximately 13 600 to 20 400 deaths. JE primarily affects children. Most adults in endemic countries have natural immunity after childhood infection, but individuals of any age may be affected. It is spread by mosquitoes. The *Culex* mosquito is the vector for transmission of Japanese encephalitis virus and this virus is a member of the family-Flaviviridae and is a single-stranded positive-sense RNA virus.

The combination of stagnant water and the close proximity of mosquitoes and birds is a risk factor for Japanese encephalitis virus disease. Pigs and wild birds serve as a reservoir for the Japanese encephalitis virus disease. Since the disease is of zoonotic significance, the symptoms in man are also to be understood (paresis, paralysis, flaccid neck, circling and tremors). There is no cure for the disease. Clearance of bushes near the water bodies in free ranging regions that accommodate the different types of water bodies to which the wild ducks of migratory types visit in the concerned seasons of the year shall be considered as the highly essential one in the prevention of the occurrence of these viral infections. Disposal of the carcasses in due time with adaptation of appropriate hygienic measures and appropriate bio-security measures have to be adapted.

It needs more intensive research to determine the précised role of aquatic birds like ducks, geese etc. related to the occurrence of Japanese encephalitis in case of homosapiens.

Botulism (Limberneck, Bulbar Paralysis, Western Sickness and Alkali Disease)

This may become a major cause of death in water fowls like ducks, in general. There are three naturally occurring forms of botulism, infant or intestinal botulism, food borne botulism, and wound botulism. Botulism is a potential lethal disease in animals as well as in human, a neuro-paralytic disease caused by *Clostridium botulinum* toxin.

The Avian Botulism is a neuro-muscular illness caused by Botulinum (natural toxin) that is produced by bacteria - *Clostridium botulinum*. The bacteria are commonly found in the soil, rivers, and seawater. It affects both humans and animals. The bacteria also need anaerobic (absence of oxygen) conditions and do not grow in acidic conditions. It affects the nervous system of birds, leading to paralysis in their legs and wings. The outbreaks of avian botulism tend to occur when average temperatures are above 21 degrees celsius and during droughts.

Etiology

This is a toxicity related disease in water fowls like the wild ducks. It is caused by the bacterial toxin that is produced by the anaerobic bacterial organism named *Clostridium botulinum,* mainly the types A and C. Eight types of *C. botulinum* (A, B, C1, C2, D, E, F, G) have been recognized, each elaborating an immunologically distinct form of toxin. Botulinum neurotoxins are the most powerful biological toxins known and, in some countries, they have been studied and developed as biological weapon. The C. botulinum is widely distributed in the soil and vegetation, intestinal contents of mammals, birds and fish.

Wild ducks may consume the decaying fish (or) other decaying fauna in water resources, including the plant wastes and generally the botulism related toxins are produced in the decaying matters as well as the plant wastes. Hence, the water fowls get affected by botulism i.e. This disease is common in the wild ducks feeding on the dead-fish and/or spoiled vegetations esp. in the shorelines of the water sources found abundant at the wildlife regions or in their migratory routes. In this context, it becomes to mention that it is the wild turkeys which are the only resistant birds for occurrence of botulism in general.

Epidemiology

About 7,000 water birds died in Lake Michigan in the year 2007 and in the year 2008. Similarly, in Hawaii, the botulinum toxin killed around 183 Laysan Ducks in 2008. Similarly, in 2019, more than 4800 migratory bird carcasses (Ruddy Shelducks were also found dead in this instance), in and around Rajasthan state's Sambhar Lake were recovered and avian botulism was confirmed as the cause of death by IVRI, UP state, subsequently. The botulism outbreaks are likely to become more frequent in many countries, due to the reason that the existing climate-change which is found at the global level due to the multi-faceted etiological factors may lead to many alterations in the existing wetland-conditions of various countries and this may often favour multiple species of bacteria and other pathogens.

Incidence

The water sources may get contaminated due to the presence of multifaceted-etiological factors and in such occasions, one can anticipate the encountering of a massive "die-off" among the wild ducks.

The incidence is mostly in water fowls that are feeding on the decayed animal or plant matter and esp. the dead fishes floating on the water bodies esp. on the stagnated water sources.

Transmission

Avian botulism, a naturally occurring neurotoxin activated in warm weather by bacteria in silt, is passed along to waterbirds through infected bugs, causing paralysis or death. Decomposed animal or bird carcasses are the source of transmission of toxins related to the botulism. Additionally, it is to be remembered that the contamination of soil and water bodies occur from the droppings of birds, in addition to the decomposing carcasses including the fish-fauna.

Pathogenesis

After toxin is absorbed, it enters the bloodstream and travels to peripheral cholinergic synapses, primarily the neuromuscular junction. Once at these sites, botulinum toxin is internalized and enzymatically prevents the release of acetyl choline leads to paralysis.

Clinical findings

The botulism in birds regardless of the species causes rapidly fatal motor paralysis. The toxins are basically the neurotoxins that are capable of producing the facial paralysis and hence, the affected bird dies due to the respiratory paralysis.

Flaccid paralysis of the legs and wings occur before the death. Per-acute cases end quickly in death. When neck muscles are affected, the head of the botulism affected birds may hang limp, thus causing a condition referred as limberneck.

It is also true that some affected birds may recover, without any treatment.

Necropsy findings

Post-mortem examinations in general may not reveal any significant pathological changes.

Diagnosis

Biological tests shall be carried out in mice; the supernatant of the centrifuged intestinal contents from the hindgut of intestinal tract shall be subjected to membrane filtration and then duly inoculated into the mice and in positive cases, the inoculation kills the mice quickly.

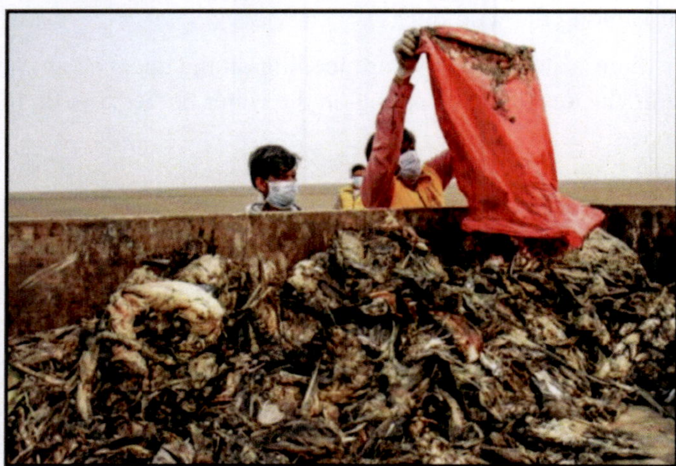

Fig 1 : Removal of bird carcasses from Sambhar Lake *(AFP Photo/Himanshu SHARMA)*

Differential diagnosis: The disease is to be differentiated from following conditions in birds-

- Spirochaetosis
- Avian duck cholera
- Other septicaemias in ducks.

Treatment

- Provision of good feed and water helps the recovery
- Trivalent (A, B, E) Botulinum Antitoxin-derived from equine sources utilizing whole antibodies (Fab and Fc portions) or Heptavalent (A, B, C, D, E, F, G) Botulinum Antitoxin-derived from "despeciated" equine IgG antibodies which have had the Fc portion cleaved off leaving the F(ab')2 portions shall be used in high-valued affected birds.

Prevention and Control

The prevention of the access to the affected carcasses or the affected decaying vegetation in the water sources has to be affected in a concrete manner. Remove the source of toxin in that area for which thorough probing is required in the concerned wildlife region.

Hygienic disposal of carcasses in water bodies regardless of the species in timely manner is highly warranted towards effecting the successful prevention of botulism in the wild ducks at free ranging regions.

The prompt removal of the fish carcasses often leads to a rapid resolution of the outbreak of the disease, highlighting the relevance of a correct method of wildlife management.

Sick birds should be captured and kept isolated and to be provided with good food and water; after recovery, they may be released in wildlife region, following the regulatory measures of the forest department, as per the Wildlife Protection Act, 1972.

Duck Pasteurellosis

(Syn: Avian Pasteurellosis/Avian Cholera in ducks, Duck cholera and Duck Haemorrhagic Septicaemia, Duck Septicaemia, New Duck Disease)

Avian cholera, a contagious disease caused by the bacterium *Pasteurella multocida,* is commonly found in both domestic poultry and migratory birds. It causes acute mortality and chronic suppurative necrosis.

Etiology

Pasteurella multocida has been found in many species of birds and mammals. *Pasteurella multocida* is considered a single species although it includes three subspecies: *multocida*, *septica*, and *gallicida*. The subspecies *multocida* is the most common cause of disease, but *septica* and *gallicida* may also cause cholera-like disease. *Pasteurella multocida* can be sub grouped by capsule serogroup antigens into five capsular types (A, B, C, D, and F) and into 16 somatic serotypes.

However, this disease is caused in ducks by *Pasteruella anatipestifer* (Syn. *Riemerella anatipestifer*) and it mostly affects growing ducklings below 8 weeks of age and is responsible for a significant mortality; many times, this duck septicaemia-infection coincides the occurrence of duck viral enteritis (duck plague).

Epidemiology

Infections with *Pasteurella multocida* (fowl cholera) in ducks are extremely common across the world. This organism is very common in Asia and the Middle East countries. Documentations are available with domestic ducks but research in wild ducks are remotely carried out, in general.

Incidence

Riemerella anatipestifer causes disease in ducks throughout the world. Formerly known as *Pasteurella anatipestifer*, this organism usually causes disease in young ducklings aged between 2 and 6 weeks. The disease is one of the commonly encountered duck diseases (both the domestic as well as the wild ducks) and often, acute types of infections are common among the ducks.

The transmission is through aerosol, feed, water and fomites; it has also been shown to be transmitted vertically through infected eggs. The bacterium is susceptible to environmental factors and general disinfectants.

Transmission

Cholera infections usually take place within 48 hours of exposure, which typically occurs through bird-to-bird contact or ingestion of contaminated food and water. In wild waterfowl, a predictable seasonal pattern exists in areas where avian cholera has become well established and is closely associated with seasonal migration patterns when birds are densely concentrated.

The causal organism of duck septicaemia is thought to be vertically transmitted through the egg and lateral transmission occurs via the respiratory route. Stress factors such as moving birds and environmental variations can trigger disease.

Chronically infected birds and asymptomatic carriers are considered to be major sources of infection. Wild birds like water fowls which include the wild ducks also may introduce the organism into a poultry flock, but mammals (including rodents, pigs, dogs, and cats) may also carry the infection.

Pathogenesis

Inflammation of pericardium with haemorrhagic areas, air sacs and gastro-intestinal tract are generally encountered as pathogenic effects in the affected birds. Respiratory system also may get involved.

Clinical findings

In ducks, fowl cholera most frequently occurs as an acute septicaemic infection, often with many acute deaths.

- Birds infected with cholera often appear lethargic and drowsy and may suffer convulsions, swim in circles, or be reluctant to fly.
- Depression, mucoid discharge from the mouth, ruffled feathers, diarrhoea, and increased respiratory rate are noticed,
- The disease is characterized by the occurrence of swollen head, wattle, joints, in addition to the foot pad.
- In acute cases, often the affected birds die quickly.

Necropsy findings

The common lesions are fibrinous pericarditis, hepatitis and air sacculitis. Parenchymatous degeneration of liver and diffuse fibrinous meningitis are also encountered.

Other lesions that can be anticipated in avian cholera are quoted below-

- Vascular regions are mainly affected as reflected by congestion and hyperaemia throughout the carcasses.
- Caseous arthritis
- Productive inflammation of the peritoneal cavity
- In sub-acute cases, common is the occurrence of the necrotic foci throughout the liver and spleen.
- In chronic cases, suppurative lesions involving respiratory tract, conjunctiva and adjacent areas of head region are commonly encountered in the affected birds.
- Sequestered necrotic lung lesions generally lead to the suspicion of haemorrhagic septicaemia in birds

Diagnosis

The disease is generally diagnosed by means of symptoms, post-mortem lesions, history of earlier occurrence in that area etc.

Demonstration of bipolar organisms in microscopic examination of blood and tissue smears is also confirmatory. Heart-blood swab from the fresh duck-carcasses is much useful for diagnostic purposes. Primary isolation can be accomplished using media such as blood agar, dextrose starch agar, or trypticase soy agar (TCA). Isolation may be improved by the addition of 5% heat-inactivated serum.

Pathogenicity test shall be done in 6-8 weeks old mice (white swiss) and the pathogenic isolates generally cause mortality in the mice within 24 hours. Isolation of organism from dead mice also may fulfil the Koch's postulates for the confirmation of the death of mice due to pasteurellosis. The stained impression smears of important organs reveal the presence of typical bipolar organism.

Serologic testing can be done by rapid whole blood agglutination, serum plate agglutination, agar diffusion tests, and ELISA. Advanced molecular diagnostic tests like PCR helps to find out these organisms.

Differential diagnosis

Other bacterial organisms causing pneumonia and peritoneal fluid accumulation need to be differentiated by means of culture, isolation and PCR.

Treatment

Treatment in free ranging wild ducks is difficult but in high valued birds, capture of diseased birds as identified by clinical symptoms and history of earlier occurrence shall be considered as one of the bases for the suspicion of this disease in the wild ducks there. Antibiotic sensitivity tests shall be performed before usage of drugs against the incidence of duck pasteurellosis and this gains significance especially during the emergence of multi-drug-resistant strains of the causal organism in the wild ducks. Sulfamethazine (or) sulfadimethoxine in feed or water shall be used carefully in order to control the mortality and penicillin shall be used in cases of resistance to the sulpha drugs. High levels of tetracycline antibiotics in the feed (0.04%), drinking water, or administered parenterally may be useful.

Chloramphenicol may be given at dose of 1 gm / 5 lit of water or 50 gm/100 kg feed along with anti-stress and hepato-protective supportive therapy, in the event of capture of wild ducks for rescue purpose if any.

Prevention and Control

- Isolation of the diseased birds
- Disposal of carcasses from water bodies immediately
- Periodic checking of birds for evidence of exposure or existence of disease by the serological testing methods etc.
- Placement of barriers in and around the water bodies, if a greater number of cases are found affected may help discourage the use of the infected resources by the wild ducks.

- Systematic follow-up of general principles pertaining to the hygiene and the biosecurity.

Salmonella Infections: Fowl Typhoid in Ducks and Pullorum (Bacillary White Diarrhoea / Salmonellosis) in Ducks

Etiology

Fowl typhoid is indistinguishable from pullorum disease unless the etiological agent is isolated and identified. The true salmonellosis is comparatively rare in ducks but is often due to the serotype *Salmonella typhimurium,* where as the Fowl typhoid and Pullorum disease are caused by two different biovars of *Salmonella enterica* subsp. Enterica serovar gallinarum, a Gram negative bacterial rod in Salmonella serogroup D (non-flagellated organisms with O antigens 1, 9 and 12) in the family Enterobacteriaceae.

Fowl typhoid

Salmonella enterica subsp. Enterica serovar gallinarum biovar gallinarum, which causes fowl typhoid, is usually abbreviated as *Salmonella gallinarum*

Pullorum (or) Bacillary white diarrhoea

Salmonella enterica subsp. Enterica serovar Gallinarum biovar Pullorum as *Salmonella pullorum.* Pullorum disease, previously known as Bacillary White Diarrhoea, in poultry is caused by *Salmonella pullorum*. Pullorum disease is generally a disease of poultry caused by the bacterium *Salmonella pullorum which is a* subspecies of the bacterium *Salmonella enterica*, which also causes human food-borne illness. This disease is characterized by white diarrhea and the mortality rate can reach 100%

Epidemiology

Incidence

The diseases of Fowl typhoid and Pullorum are most often observed in captive chickens, turkeys and also in the game birds like pheasants, quail, guinea fowl, partridges, peacocks etc. Either one (or) both of these organisms have been additionally reported in the ducks, geese, various psittacines, sparrows, starlings etc.

Transmission

In fowl typhoid, faecal-oral contamination becomes the major mode of transmission and trans-ovarian transmission is also possible. Carriers are possible with in Salmonella organism based infections in general. Pullorum disease is spread from infected parent birds via the egg to the new-born bird.

Pathogenesis

In Fowl typhoid, inflammatory changes are seen along with the necrotic changes thus interfering with the liver functions in wild ducks. Spleen and kidneys also get inflamed additionally.

In Bacillary white diarrhoea, subsequent to the invasion of bacterial organisms, there are inflammatory cells coupled with exudation leading to severe diarrhoea in the affected birds. Endo-toxins are produced and disseminated intra-vascular coagulation (DIC) along with micro-vasculature failure may occur leading to shock and death in the affected birds.

Clinical findings

The clinical signs of Fowl typhoid as well as Pullorum disease in aves are similar in nature, esp. In the younger birds; older birds may become pale, dehydrated, and have diarrhoea.

The Fowl typhoid disease is characterized by the occurrence of swollen head, wattle, joints, in addition to the foot pad-involvement.

However, in Pullorum or Bacillary white diarrhoea, the affected ducks reveal whitish diarrhoea along with respiratory distress and drooped wings; in less acute cases, nervous signs along with the swollen joints are encountered. Many times, in Pullorum disease, symptoms esp. in adult birds may not be apparent.

Necropsy findings

In Fowl typhoid

The Fowl typhoid affected aves overall may reveal the following significant post mortem lesions and changes, in the affected birds.

- Swollen, friable, and often bile-stained liver, with or without necrotic foci
- Enlargement of spleen
- Swollen kidney
- Anemia
- Enteritis

In Pullorum(or) Bacillary white diarrhoea

- Pale areas in myocardium and gizzard muscles
- Splenic enlargement, with congestion
- Yellow coloured liver with haemorrhagic streaks
- Sero-fibrinous pericarditis and peritonitis
- Enlargement of kidney

Diagnosis

Fowl typhoid

The disease is possible by means of systematic confirmation by isolation, identification, and serotyping of the causal organisms of Fowl typhoid as well as Pullorum. In addition to serology, ELISA, Tube agglutination and Rapid whole blood agglutination are helpful in diagnosis of Fowl typhoid.

Pullorum (or) Bacillary white diarrhoea

Enrichment and selective media may be sued for isolation of the organisms.

Detection of antibodies in the suspected group of ducks shall be made by the whole blood agglutination test

Differential diagnosis

This disease should be differentiated with diseases of similar clinical signs and symptoms like pasteurellosis, colibacillosis, duck viral enteritis etc.

Treatment

The affected birds shall be isolated and treated with broad-spectrum antibiotics on daily basis for a week period.

Prevention and Control

These are practically difficult and in severe incidences, prevention of access to the contaminated water source may be helpful to a great extent.

Regular check to avoid sewage water-based contamination of the wet lands to avoid occurrence of bacterial infections like salmonellosis among the waterfowls that include the wild ducks also.

Colibacillosis

Avian colibacillosis is an infectious disease of birds caused by *Escherichia coli*, which is considered as one of the principal causes of morbidity and mortality. Birds of all species and age groups get affected by these organisms.

Etiology

Escherichia coli cause the infection in ducks, as the case with many species of the birds.

Incidence

- This is by far the most common bacterial infection of all ages of commercial ducks than the wild ducks. However, being an environmental organism, it can act as a primary causal organism or secondary to other infections such as viruses in water fowls.

- Young and growing birds are highly affected.

Transmission

The *E. coli* is mainly transmitted by faeco-oral route and any secretions or excretion from the body may act as a source of infections to susceptible birds.

Pathogenesis

- Inflammation of the intestinal tract is the major pathogenic effect
- Emaciation may be seen in the ducks
- Following invasion through the intestinal mucosa, cecal tonsils and Peyer's patches, the organisms are engulfed by macrophages, and through the blood stream and/or lymphatic systems, they spread to organs rich in reticulo-endothelial tissues (RES), such as liver and spleen, which are the main sites of multiplication

Clinical findings

Signs in affected birds can vary from sudden death to birds being 'off-colour' with their necks pulled into their bodies. Severe diarrhoea is evident and below the tail region, watery dropping stained appearance may be noticed in long-time land-wandering/standing ducks, near the water sources.

Necropsy findings

The necropsy findings in ducks are almost similar to the turkeys (or) fowls. Congestion of lungs with haemorrhages of heart and air sacs. More chronic infections will reveal the characteristic lesions of pericarditis, peri-hepatitis, enlargement of the liver, air sacculitis and pneumonia.

Diagnosis

Diagnosis is relatively straight forward, based on the post mortem findings and a rapid growth of the organism on blood or MacConkey agar.

Differential diagnosis

The disease is to be differentiated from other bacterial infection-based diarrhoea and isolation and identification of the organism shall be carried out for differential diagnosis, from the available stool samples, intestinal contents etc. of the wild ducks.

Further, serological tests including ELISA and molecular diagnostic tests like PCR will be helpful in precise identification of the organism.

Treatment

Antibiotic sensitivity tests need to be performed and accordingly the therapy shall be undertaken in captured birds that are found to be affected at water sources.

Prevention and Control

The prevention of the access to the affected water sources shall be attempted in the event of die-offs among water fowls including the wild ducks. Remove the dead birds immediately from the water bodies if found.

Hygienic disposal of carcasses in water bodies regardless of the species in timely manner is highly warranted towards effecting the successful prevention of botulism in the wild ducks at free ranging regions.

The prompt removal of the fish carcasses often leads to a rapid resolution of the outbreak of the disease, highlighting the relevance of a correct method of wildlife management. Sick birds should be captured and kept isolated and to be provided with good food and water; after recovery, they may be released in wildlife region, following the regulatory measures of the forest department, as per the Wildlife Protection Act, 1972.

Streptococcal Infections

Increased levels of mortality at around 10 to 14 days of age in commercial duck flocks associated with poor hygiene have been implicated with infection by *Streptococcus zooepidemicus* and the post-mortem findings include congested carcasses, enlarged and mottled spleens and often air sacculitis. However, documentations in wild ducks are scarce.

References

Adames, A.J., Dutary, B., Tejera, H., Adames, E. and Galindo, P. (1993). The relationship between mosquito vectors and aquatic birds in the potential transmission of 2 arboviruses. Rev. Med. Panama.18(2)106-119.

Adhya, D., Dutta, K. and Basu, A. (2013) Japanese encephalitis in India: risk of an epidemic in the National Capital Region. International Health. 5(3)166-168.

Communication of Iowa State University. College of Veterinary Medicine.Fowl Typhoid and Pullorum Disease Bacillary White Diarrhea (Pullorum Disease). January, 2019.

Cova, L., Lambert, V.R., Chevallier, A., Hantz, O., Fourel, I., Jacquet, L.C., Pichoud, C., Boulay, J., Chomel, B., Vitvitski, L. and Trepo, C. (1986). Evidence for the Presence of Duck Hepatitis B Virus in Wild Migrating Ducks. J. gen. Virol. 67:537-547.

Dhama, K., Kumar, N., Saminathan, M., Tiwari, R., Karthik, K., Kumar, A., Palanivelu, M., Shabbir, M.Z., Malik, Y.Z. and Singh, R.K. (2014). Epiedmiology of Duck Viral Enteritis. DOI: 10.2478/bvip-2014-0078

Eldin, W. F. S. and Reda, L. M. Epidemiological prevalence of Pasteurell-amultocida in ducks. (2016). Japanese Journal of Veterinary Research. 64(2)251-255. Kozdruń, W., Czekaj, H. and Lorek, M. Outbreak of duck viral hepatitis in duckling flocks in Poland. Bull Vet Inst Pulawy. 58:513-515.

Maity, D.K., Chatterjee, A., Guha, C. and Biswas, U. (2012). Pasteurellosis in Duck In West Bengal. Explor. Anim. Med. Res., 1(2)119-123

Mizzima Foundation News. (2019). Botulism feared responsible for India migratory bird deaths.

Mohan, K. and Kumar, P.G.P., Pasteurellosis in a duck. Veterinary World. 1(12):367

Punnoose, P., Vineetha S. and M. Mahesh. (2021). Current scenario and pathology of duck diseases - A systematic review. Indian J. Vet.Path. 45(4):242-265.

USGS Avian Cholera. (2013). USGS Field Manual of Wildlife Diseases: Birds.

Vov, LDK and Vov. Role of birds in importing and preserving arboviruses. 1974. 43(4)473-480.

WHO. Epidemiology of Avian Influenza. Agriculture Department. Animal Production and Health Division.

WHO Report on Influenza (Avian and other zoonotic diseases)

Wobeser, G.A., Diseases of Wild Waterfowl. 1997

14

Economics of Duck Rearing

In this chapter we will discuss about economics of raising 100 Khaki Campbell duck for egg production. Popular breed of ducks for egg production includes Khaki Campbell and Indian Runner. Among the egg laying breeds, Khaki Campbell is the best producer. Individual egg production of almost an egg a day in this breed for well over twelve months has been recorded and flock averages in excess of 300 eggs per duck per year are not uncommon. Khaki Campbell ducks weigh about 2-2.2 kgs and drakes 2.2-2.4 kgs. Egg size varies from 65-70 gms.

Cost and estimates for establishment of a 100+15 Khaki Campbell duck unit (under semi-intensive system)

S. No.	Particulars	Amount (Rs.)
1.	Shed/Enclosures for 100+15 duck for 50 sq. ft. @ ₹ 20/ per sq. ft.	₹ 10,000.00
2.	Accessories viz. light, feederer, waterer, laying boxes, buckets @ ₹ 5/ duck	₹ 575.00
3.	Cost of ducklings (115+6 assuming 5% mortality) @ ₹ 35 per duckling	₹ 4,235.00
4.	Feed cost for initial 6 months (9 kg per bird @ ₹ 15/kg)	₹ 15,525.00
5.	Other miscellaneous cost including insurance cost etc.	₹ 675.00
6.	Total cost involved	₹ 31,010.00
7.	Margin (Own contribution)	₹ 0.00
8.	Bank Loan	₹ 31,010.00
	Say ₹	₹ 31,000.00

S. No.	Particulars	Years		
A. Recurring expenditure		1	2	3
1.	Feed cost (1-6 months-9 kg per bird; 6-12th months – 12 kg per bird; 2nd year- 24 kg per bird; 3rd year onwards – 25 kg per bird) @ ₹ 15.00 per kg.	₹ 36225	₹ 41400	₹ 41400

2.	Cost of medicine and vaccination (1st year- ₹ 2/- per bird; 2nd year onwards- ₹ 4/- per bird)	₹ 230	₹ 460	₹ 460
3.	Labour (@ ₹ 0/- per day- self-employment)	₹ 0	₹ 0	₹ 0
Total		₹ 36455	₹ 41860	₹ 41860
B. Income				
1.	Sale of eggs 9250 eggs/bird @ ₹ 4/- per egg)	₹ 80000	₹ 10000	₹ 10000
2.	Sale of culled ducks (1.8 kg/bird @ ₹ 120/- per kg)	₹ 0	₹ 0	₹ 24840
3.	Sale of manure @ ₹ 20 per bird	₹ 1150	₹ 2300	₹ 2300
Gross income		₹ 81150	₹ 102300	₹ 127140
4. Depreciation of shed @ 10.00%		₹ 1000	₹ 1000.00	₹ 1000.00
5. Depreciation of equipment @ 15.00%		₹ 86.00	₹ 86.00	₹ 86.00
Net profit		₹ 43,609	₹ 59,354	₹ 84,194

Year	**Bank Loan**	**Gross Surplus**	**Repayment**		**Total**	**Net Surplus**
			Principal	**Interest**		
I	₹ 31000	₹ 43609	₹ 10333	₹ 3720	₹ 14053	₹ 29556
II	₹ 20667	₹ 59354	₹ 10333	₹ 2480	₹ 12813	₹ 46541
III	₹ 10334	₹ 84194	₹ 10334	₹ 1240	₹ 11574	₹ 72620

Unit cost, Bank loan estimate for a Duck rearing unit of 100 Ducks + 15 Drakes

1. Shed/enclosures for 100 + 15 duck for 500 sq. ft @ ₹ 20/- per sq.ft	₹ 10000
2. Duck feeding, watering and egg laying boxes, buckets etc lumpsum	₹ 1500
3. Duck lings 3 months old 115 + 15 i.e. 130 @ ₹ 130/- per duck (including transport loss)	₹ 16900
4. Feed cost for first 2 months during growing of one month and one month of initial laying period @ 1.5 kg + 2 kg = 3.5 kg per bird @ ₹ 7/- per kg	₹ 3185
5 Cost of medicines and vaccination	₹ 1500
6 Other misc. cost including insurance cost etc. lump-sum	₹ 675
Total cost	₹ 33760
Say Total cost	₹ 34000
Margin money @5.00% of total cost	₹ 2000
Bank loan	₹ 32000

Production chart

S. No.	Particulars	1 Year		2 Year		3 Year		4 Year	
		1 to 6	**7 to 12**	**1 to 6**	**7 to 12**	**1 to6**	**7 to 12**	**1 to 6**	**7 to 12**
1	Purchase of duck lings (3 months old)	100+15	----					100+15 (2nd batch)	
2	Growing	100 + 15						100+15	
3	Laying	100 (5 & 6 month)	100	100	100	100	100	100 (1st batch- 4months) (2nd batch - 2 months)	100 (2nd batch)
4	Culling	---						105	

Economics / Cash flow statement of 100 + 15 Duck unit

S. No.	Particulars	Year				
Recurring cost		1	2	3	4	5
1	Feed cost for adult ducks	9,660	19,320	19,320	20,125	20,125
2	Feed cost for young duck lings	----	-----	-----	7,245	-----
3	Medicine cost	230	460	460	460	460
4	Other misc cost	500	500	500	500	500
5	Cost of duck lings	----	----	----	1,725	----
	Total recurring cost	10,390	20,280	20,280	30,055	21,085
Sale receipt						
1	Sale of eggs	40,000	60,000	60,000	60,000	60,000
2	Sale of culled ducks	----	----	----	4,725	----
3	Sale of manure	575	1,150	1,150	1,150	1,150
	Total Benefits	40,575	61,150	61,150	65,875	61,150
	Gross Surplus	30,185	40,870	40,870	35,820	40,065

Loan repayment for 100 + 15 Duck unit

Year	Bank loan	Gross surplus	Repayment		Total	Net surplus
			Principle	Interest		
I	32,000	30,185	6,400	3,840	10,240	19,945
II	25,600	40,870	6,400	3,072	9,472	31,398
III	19,200	40,870	6,400	2,304	8,704	32,166
IV	12,800	35,820	6,400	1,536	7,936	27,884
V	6,400	40,065	6,400	768	7,168	32,897

Remarks

The figure given are purely for reference and it may very from region to region. For any entrepreneur would like to study for sustainability the above model may fellow.

Index

L

M

N

O

P